HOW TO CURE
MYOFASCIAL PAIN

HOW TO CURE MYOFASCIAL PAIN

Pentti Raaste MD.

authorHOUSE®

AuthorHouse™ UK Ltd.
1663 Liberty Drive
Bloomington, IN 47403 USA
www.authorhouse.co.uk
Phone: 0800.197.4150

The information, ideas, and suggestions in this book are not intended as a substitute for professional medical advice. Before following any suggestions contained in this book, you should consult your personal physician. Neither the author nor the publisher shall be liable or responsible for any loss or damage allegedly arising as a consequence of your use or application of any information or suggestions in this book.

Published by AuthorHouse   05/21/2013

ISBN: 978-1-4817-9598-2 (sc)
ISBN: 978-1-4817-9599-9 (hc)
ISBN: 978-1-4817-9600-2 (e)

Library of Congress Control Number: 2013909340

Any people depicted in stock imagery provided by Thinkstock are models, and such images are being used for illustrative purposes only.
Certain stock imagery © Thinkstock.

This book is printed on acid-free paper.

Because of the dynamic nature of the Internet, any web addresses or links contained in this book may have changed since publication and may no longer be valid. The views expressed in this work are solely those of the author and do not necessarily reflect the views of the publisher, and the publisher hereby disclaims any responsibility for them.

CONTENTS

INTRODUCTION

My interest in pain relief treatment began before graduating. During my last years of study, I worked long hours on multiple sites, in outpatient and in accident and emergency, covering shifts. Back pain in particular was a challenge to treat, because the treatment regimes we had studied did not seem to work. We treated with medication, signing the patient off sick, rest, and physiotherapy. Patients kept returning, and no matter how we treated them, the pain was still present. For a young doctor with great enthusiasm, it was disheartening and created a feeling of failure, anger, and helplessness.

Some disgruntled patients prompted me to embark on a search to find other techniques and increase my tool box of items for relieving pain. They returned to my office simply to inform me that doctors were of little help, so they had gone to visit a healer or a chiropractor and were now completely cured! Of course it was hard to hear, but I thought, "Why do chiropractors know more than a doctor initiated into the secrets of the human body?" I wanted to learn, and so I started to study different paramedical techniques. I have to thank the patients whose difficulties I found challenging.

One of my first teachers was a Norwegian neurologist, Professor Henrik Seyffarth. Seyffarth was well-known in his home country at the time as the author of several scientific papers and popular books such as "Relax and You Will Be Cured". He participated in radio programmes and even had his own magazine. He developed his version of Dr Huneke's neural therapy. Seyffarth infiltrated areas of greatest pain and stiffness in muscles with dilute procaine (local anaesthetic) in fairly large quantities. He called the sites of pain myosis, now known as trigger points. It was discovered that these areas were hardened areas of muscle with ischemia. Dr Seyffarth advised that the source of pain was not always found in the area where the patient felt pain; the pain could radiate fairly long distances. In addition, he devoted much attention to the possible causes of pain and malfunction, correcting poor posture and ergonomics.

I worked in Seyffarth's office for some time and studied his technique. I also read his books and articles. In my opinion, the best way to learn was to observe practice. Many of his explanations are still valid today.

When I was desperately looking for some treatment for my daughter, who was seriously ill, I found a doctor who practiced homeopathy and acupuncture in Finland. In 1972, he was the only and the first to practice those techniques in Finland. These treatments were not accepted at that time in medical circles, but he encouraged me to study acupuncture and explained the benefits of the method. I contacted the physician and acupuncturist Dr Felix Mann in London, and I participated in one of his courses in 1973 and learned a valuable new technique to my arsenal against pain and other diseases. Most acupuncture points coincide with the trigger points and other key points in the treatment of musculoskeletal pain (myofascial pain). It was a technique rejected by official medicine at that time, but now, thirty-five years later, it has become a part of medicine and is taught to medical and physiotherapy students.

The same year I signed up for a course that was given by Norwegian physiotherapists in Finland called "manual therapy of the dorsal spine no. 1", or "manual orthopaedic treatment" (OMT). The course covered different chiropractic techniques, and I had already had several patients who were cured with the help of chiropractors in a way that seemed miraculous to me. I had high hopes for the success of these innovating techniques. The course was very interesting but it only covered a small part. Then in 1976, I had the opportunity to join the University of Ulleval in Oslo, under Professor Asbjørn Bragstad, to continue and complete my studies in manual therapy. I was the only doctor in the group; the rest were all physiotherapists. I participated for almost two years and learned a thorough diagnosis of the musculoskeletal system—details of each joint, its anatomy and function. It was very valuable knowledge and was far more detailed than I was taught in medical school.

In one of my visits to London, I contacted and visited a well-known physician, osteopath, and author, Dr Allan Stoddard. His way of working was very similar to what I had studied in Norway. I also studied other well-known authors such as Dr Cyriax and Dr Lindh. (The Swedish doctor Lindh based her PhD on the method called "auto traction".)

Manipulation techniques were quite efficient in certain cases; however, it did surprise me that the method concentrated solely on the joints and their movements, not taking into account the muscles and other soft tissues surrounding the joint. Even before the "manipulative" studies, I had learned some massage techniques. I began practicing deep muscle massage techniques, which was a long-standing tradition in Finland that combined sauna and massage. The heat of the sauna increases circulation, as well as relaxes and preheats the body before massage. (Now instead, physiotherapists use various devices to warm and relax the tissues.) Finish massage therapists treated many ailments and had learned to locate the muscles that were hurting and needed massage. They would spend more than two hours for a full-body massage, and their treatments were quite effective. They had no formal education but learnt from experience. Massage was often carried out as a family tradition. Unfortunately this tradition is gradually being lost.

I also studied other massage techniques that are necessary for different problems, such as lymphatic drainage massage, connective tissue massage, acupressure, reflexology, Dr Furter's technique, and others.

Radiation of pain remains a mystery. Pain may radiate upwards or downwards. The mystery is that it does not follow the anatomy of nerves. Doctors such as Verne and JH Kellgren have done studies on the subject. The mystery is still there because the pain does not necessarily radiate equally in different patients, and we do not know why.

With years of practice and after having the opportunity to compare in practice the effectiveness of different techniques, I want to share my conclusions in this book. The theory is, in my opinion, well covered by literature; in particular, the book by Travell and Simons is very comprehensive and covers much of the research that has been done in this field. Another great book is by Dr Clair Davies, *The Trigger Point Therapy Workbook*. Dr Devin Starlanyl suffers herself of both fibromyalgia and myofascial pain. Her book includes her own experience and is called *Fibromyalgia and Chronic Myofascial Pain*.

In my book, I do not only talk about the trigger points but also about other painful sites that do not have the same exact definition as defined by Travell and Simons. In my opinion, one has to treat all painful sites, including in the tendons and joint capsules.

This book is primarily addressed to professionals, but even patients can find hints on how to help themselves. Many areas can be treated to some extent by the patient himself. The injections or punctures make the treatment more effective, but one can accomplish many things without them only with an effective massage. Who is better than the patient himself to find the points of maximum pain and massage them? The massage must feel a bit painful in order to be efficient. If one feels soreness afterwards, let the site rest a couple of days and then continue the treatment. This treatment can save unnecessary suffering and also significantly reduce economic loss on sick leave and disability benefits, medicines, and other treatments.

2. REASONS AND MY THANKS

I have a desire to share my knowledge and my effective treatment methods with practitioners and patients so that they can request it. Furthermore, the instructions in this booklet may also serve as a self-help guide. The myofascial pains are the most common types of pain. It is estimated that 60-70 per cent of all pain is of myofascial origin. Although it is not life threatening, it reduces quality of life and the functional capacity of the body, and it can cause many unnecessary expenses. These pains can often be completely cured with the appropriate treatment.

I like professionals to be able to adapt this method by reading and understanding this book and using the technique shown in my companion DVD. A physical therapist or masseuse can greatly improve his performance by concentrating treatment in the myofascial trigger points, and even more so by using the technique of dry needling. The best option would be to work together with a doctor who knows how to infiltrate the points. With the combination of the infiltration techniques, I have achieved the best and most long-lasting results.

I want to express my gratitude to my patients, from whom I continually learn new things. They have been the inspiration behind this treatment method. To all my past teachers. To Univadis, for allowing the use of their anatomical images, and to Rikke Stockwell and Nina Jarlov for helping me with the English language, and finally to AuthorHouse team for the professional editing.

3. DOUBLE-BLIND SCIENTIFIC STUDIES OR EVIDENCE-BASED MEDICINE

In the current practice of medicine, no treatment appears to have any value without scientific studies, which fill strict criteria and have a very large number of patients. For certain things, this is well and good, but despite these rigorously and well-done studies, one cannot control all the influencing factors, and for that reason the results change and the treatment recommendations are continuously changing; there is always some insecurity.

I will give just one example of these puzzling alterations: recommendations of the post-menopausal hormonal treatment (HRT), which in the beginning were recommended to all women as a miracle anti-aging method. Now, the current recommendation is to take the smallest possible dose for shortest time possible, and only if there are symptoms.

In the field of myofascial pain, it is extremely difficult to do double-blind studies. It is almost impossible to find patients who are completely identical in their suffering and thus who are comparable for the treatment results. Back pain can have very different backgrounds and be caused by any of the various existing tissues, making it impossible to compare different patients. Treatment of a prolapsed disc must be different from a sprain of a muscle or tendon. The results of treatment by manual methods are not only influenced by the method itself, but also by the therapist's personal skills. An example would be treatment with acupuncture, which may be more or less successful depending of the election of the points from the several thousand possibilities. The treatment is individual; we have to look for the evidence in different ways.

It is perhaps better to conduct studies measuring the results. Studies are needed to compare different treatment methods and therapists in their efficiency. The cost and effectiveness of different treatments is very important. There is a huge difference between classical medical treatment and physiotherapy, and these new methods of treatment of the trigger points. In my practice, I see patients who have spent months and even years on treatment with drugs, or who have had over twenty traditional physiotherapy sessions without essential success—and their pain may disappear in three to seven sessions with these innovative therapies. The advantages are clear: savings on medication and treatment costs, as well as less sick leave and improved quality of life.

4. SOME EXAMPLES OF DIFFICULT CASES, TO GIVE HOPE

1. Female, fifty-five years old.

She worked as a nurse in Finland and spent many hours standing, walking, and lifting patients. She had chronic pain in the lumbar region that she thought could not be treated further, because she had tried many different treatments without any results. She fell on her right knee a year and half ago, and since then she also had pain in the popliteal area, and the knee swelled up. She had seen many specialists and had taken anti-inflammatory drugs. An orthopaedic surgeon advised to operate, even if nothing concrete could be seen in the X-ray images. It had become worse lately, and she could barely walk.

In the examination, I found the knee joint with some hydrops, but it was stable with a strong periarthritis. She had painful points (trigger points) below and above the patella on the medial and lateral ligaments and in the popliteal area. In addition, the thigh muscles were tense and very painful with pressure. With fifteen sessions using steroid injections, transcutaneous nerve stimulator (TNS) and massage to deactivate the sore spots, she could move without pain, and the hydrops disappeared.

On her next visit to Spain, I treated her back pain. She had had her back pain for many years; the X-ray showed moderate osteoarthritis. She had sore spots at the dorsal intervertebral ligament (especially the L4-5) and at both gluteal areas, especially near the sacro-iliac joint. With five treatments using injections (corticosteroid at the worst points), TNS, and massage, she was released from her pain.

2. Male, fifty-nine years old

Seven years ago, he started having pain in his hip after some occasional long walks. He had an X-ray five years ago, and there were some signs of early osteoarthritis (first degree). He was prescribed anti-inflammatory medicine called Etoricoxib. Despite the medication, the pain increased. Four months before coming to my practice, he had an IMR scan where nothing special was found. He was in pain at night and could not sleep on the painful side.

My examination showed that the joint had good mobility, without the typical rigidity of advanced osteoarthritis. Examination of the circulation and the nerve function showed normal results. He had active trigger points in the vastus lateralis and the iliotibial tract (see photo). Other points were found in the gluteal area, especially near the sciatic tuberosity.

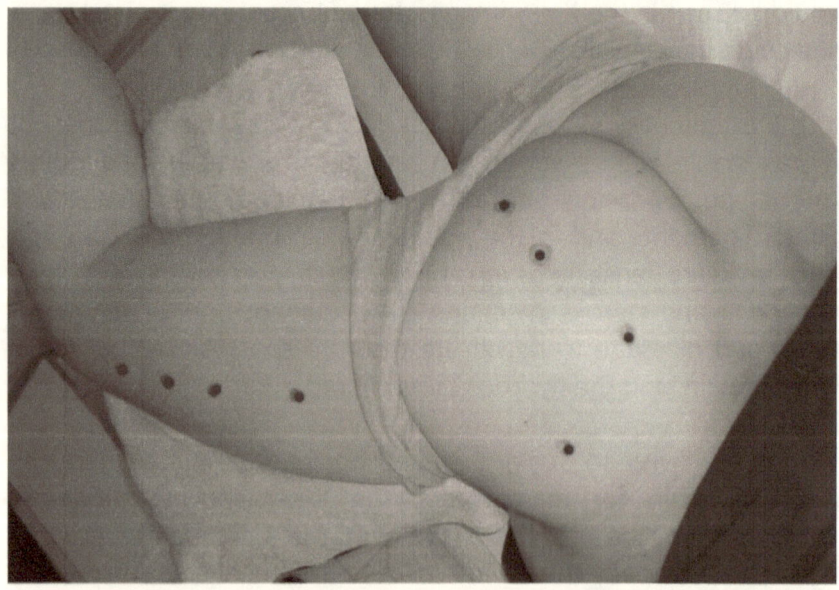

The treatment involved the usual injections of lidocaine, infrared laser to the points, and massage. With five sessions the pain was gone; he could walk without problems and had no pain while sleeping.

3. Male, fifty-eight years old

He had suffered ten years from neck pain that radiated to his head. It had lately worsened, which was the reason why he came to my practice.

My first observation was his poor posture. The radiograph showed osteoarthritis, grade one to two. There were no trapped nerves. He had sore spots in his upper back muscles, and they had a hard consistency and were contracted. The trapezius muscles and the neck muscles felt the same.

The treatment was with lidocaine injections, TNS, massage, and mobilization of the thoracic spine. After three sessions the patient felt well and without pain. I advised him on correct postures and methods of biofeedback. He corrected his posture and learned to relax the muscles in order to prevent relapses.

4. Male, sixty-five years old

When falling from a ladder, he grabbed the railing with his right hand, and his shoulder received a strong jerk. The X-rays were normal, but the shoulder began to hurt more and more. Immobilization and anti-inflammatory medicines did not improve the problem. Six months later, he visited an orthopaedic surgeon, who suggested surgery because the shoulder was now in real pain, the mobility was very much reduced, and it ached even at night. There was a suspected rupture of the rotator cuff, and a decision was made to operate. At the operation the surgeon found no rupture, but he saw a synovitis and a subacromial bursitis. The surgeon carried out an acromioplasty and a manipulation under anaesthesia in order to increase the movement range. Then the patient was prescribed rehabilitation with a physiotherapist.

Again he had a lot of pain and was developing a frozen shoulder despite the rehabilitation treatment. Six to seven weeks after the operation, he came to my practice. He had sore areas and contracture in the supraspinatus muscle, the pectoral muscles, and the scapular region (The infraspinatus and teres muscles), and even the subscapularis muscle. The internal and external rotations were reduced to forty degrees equally as the elevation of the arm.

The treatment began with corticosteroid infiltrations, infrared laser, and massage. I instructed progressive stretching exercises done at home two to three times a day, and then a weekly treatment sessions with me. In the fourth session I suppressed the corticosteroid and infiltrated with only lidocaine. After two more treatments the patient hardly felt any pain, except when he did his stretching exercises. Then he continued with his exercises at home and only had one more session with me in the next five weeks. He had no pain anymore, but he still had a small remaining restriction in the interior rotation.

5.   *Male, sixty-five years old*

He was a practitioner of sports, especially cycling. He never took care to warm the muscles up or stretch, or anything else for functional maintenance. Four months before he came to me, he started having pain in his left knee, first on the lateral side; the knee started to swell. The radiograph demonstrated mild osteoarthritis.

In my examination, I found the knee stable, and stretching of the lateral ligaments was painless. The bending was painful and missing thirty degrees of maximum flexion. He had sore areas in the rectus femoris tendon and the patellar ligament, as well as in the medial and lateral retinacula, in the rectus femoris muscle and the vastus medialis, in the fibular collateral ligament, and in the semimembranosus and semitendinosus muscles, especially at the distal end.

The treatment involved injections of lidocaine and diluted corticosteroid, TNS, and massage. At the beginning of the treatment, almost absolute rest of the knee was required. With nine treatments, one per week, the pain was gone and the knee had regained normal function with full range of movement.

5. THE PAINFUL AREAS (TRIGGER POINTS)

In this chapter we are talking of trigger points (TP) and their treatment. The treatment is also called inactivation of TPs. Previously other names and descriptions have been used for these painful spots. These conditions were called muscular rheumatism, fibrositis, myosis, induration, and muscle contractions. It was also already known that pain could radiate, although perhaps it was Dr Kellgren who first demonstrated this experimentally. The person who named the term "trigger point" for the first time was Dr Travell in 1942.

What follows are the diagnostic criteria of a trigger point in the muscles, from the book by Travell and Simons, *Myofascial Pain and Dysfunction.*

Essential criteria:

1. A history of sudden onset during or shortly following acute overload of stress, or a history of gradual onset with chronic overload of the affected muscle.

2. A taut, palpable band in the affected muscle.

3. Exquisite focal tenderness to digital pressure in the band of taut muscle fibres.

4. The patient recognises his typical pain when the sensible nodule is pressed. (Active TP)

5. The mobility range with passive stretching is reduced because of pain.

6. There are characteristic patterns of pain that are referred from trigger points, and they are specific to individual muscles.

7. Tactile or visual identification of a local spasm response elicited through snapping, palpating or needling of the tender spot.

8. Spontaneous electric activity that can be demonstrated with electromyography.

There is sometimes a characteristic referred pain, and even a local twitch response, but it does not occur for all patients. The trigger points have also been demonstrated physically. For example, one can see tiny nodules of contraction in the electron microscope. Spontaneous electrical activity is also measurable at these points, and they have certain biochemical alterations.

6. THE MOST FREQUENT CAUSES AND MECHANISMS OF MYOFASCIAL PAIN

The different causes of myofascial pain can be divided into seven groups.

1. Trauma and post-traumatic pain. Bruises and sprains cause ruptures of muscle fibres or tendons or joint capsules, with their inflammatory reactions, and healing sometimes is only partial or too slow; the injured areas continue to be inflamed and tolerate very little use.

2. Mini traumas, which often occur in tennis or golf players. The swings cause repeated jerks at the same site, and it gets inflamed.

3. Tissue overload when doing monotonous jobs or having excessive workload. In these cases, the muscles do not have enough rest to be able to return to their normal, relaxed state, and they cannot get rid of the metabolites accumulated during the exercise; this is well-known by the athletes. They need help in the form of massage, to pump the muscles and stimulate relaxation and metabolism. The same thing happens in everyday life, only in a slower tempo. Muscles can take years to gradually become blocked. The tension and the metabolites accumulate slowly and gradually begin to ache and hurt. This occurs even more when untrained muscles, not habituated, undergo sudden large burdens. Some examples: To clean all the windows of a house in one go 1-2 times a year. To paint walls or other large surfaces (when you are not a painter). To carry and lift heavy suitcases. To cut shrubs with garden shears. To lift furniture, gas bottles, or other heavy things. Suddenly walking too much when the body is not accustomed to exercise of this kind.

4. The metabolism of soft tissues (muscles and tendons) relies heavily on movement and relaxation. Prolonged tension (static), even with minimal forces involved, blocks the flow of fluids in the muscles and tendons. Finally the accumulated metabolites begin to irritate the nerve endings. Examples:

   · Poor and tense working postures, for example with the computer (tension in the arms or neck)

   · Support books or newspapers with the arms or to knit

   · Hours in the car driving

   · Nervous habits such as to tense the shoulders or to clench the teeth during sleep (bruxism)

   · Inflammation (rheumatoid arthritis, gout, arthritis, tendinitis, bursitis)

6. Stress and psychological tension. Psychological stress can cause us to tense muscles in any part of the body, even without being aware.

7. Immobility by immobilization treatment (a plaster) by pain or by lack of exercise or stretching.

The General Mechanism

The different causes I have mentioned above result in chemical changes in the tissues, with the consequent irritation of the pain nerve endings.

Painful areas have altered metabolism. They do not receive enough nutrients and oxygen and the metabolic products as lactic acid do not leave. The chemical changes maintain the condition in a rigor mortis type of contraction and the tissue does not usually cure on its own.

The accumulated metabolites or injuries sometimes cause some inflammatory reaction and fluid accumulation. Inflammation and swelling is largely around the ligaments, joint capsules and bursas and not normally around the muscle tissue. The muscle does not inflame in the same way, but rather develops contractures except in cases of muscle rupture. When there is a tendinitis, there is a need to examine the whole functional unit, because often the corresponding muscles are also affected and the whole unit needs to be treated. A contracted muscle also tenses the tendon, which results this to become affected.

In order to get long-term results with the pain treatment it is needed to discover the causes of the condition for each particular case and try to correct them.

Although trauma is a very different mechanism, the treatment procedure is similar. The treatment needs to stop the inflammation and re-establish the tissue function.

Tissues, that have been overloaded and have their function altered are more susceptible to trauma and do not tolerate as much as the tissue which is in a perfect condition.

7. THE DIAGNOSTIC PROCESS

The examination of patients with pain must be systematic. First of all, carry out a medical check-up to rule out any diseases or tumours. It is good practice to take at least one basic blood analysis and some X-rays. It is also necessary to carry out a neurological and vascular examination.

The examination of myofascial pain may start by asking the patient about what happened: how and when did the pain start? The patient history may often give the diagnosis directly. Afterwards, ask the patient to show the exact sites of pain and to demonstrate the painful movements or postures and the range of movements that he can or cannot do. Then conduct an inspection of the area itself, looking for deformities, pathological postures, swellings, muscular atrophy, pigmentary changes, and so on.

Examine the passive mobility—the movements limited by pain and compared to the normal mobility of the joint in question. In the neck it is very common to find painful limitation of lateral flexion (contraction of the scalene muscles). In the shoulder there is the typical painful arch caused by the tendinitis of the supraspinatus or the restrictions of a frozen shoulder. Restrictions in the rotation of the hip could indicate possible osteoarthritis and so on.

It is vital to assess the muscle strength. Do a manual, basic neurological examination in order to distinguish pain of neurological origin. Test for hypoesthesia, for hyperesthesia, and for the compression of the cervical and lumbar nerves. Check the peripheral arterial circulation, especially in the calf area, where the pain may be caused by limited arterial blood flow.

Remember that no imaging study can show the myofascial pain sites—the only way is still by manual palpation techniques. The whole painful area must be palpated carefully in order to find the points of maximal pain. The painful muscle points in the muscles often feel as taut bands or as indurations (see chapter four, "Trigger Points"). There are also tender points in tendons and around joints.

There is a valuable aid for diagnosis: the diagnostic local anaesthesia! This is extremely useful when we have doubts of the tissue causing the pain. Unfortunately, this technique has fallen into the sack of oblivion. Anesthetize the exact site which you think may be causing the pain. If you are right, the pain subsides. If you did not succeed, the pain remains the same, and so you have to try another location.

8. ABOUT THE TREATMENT IN GENERAL

Currently there are many different methods of pain treatment, especially using so-called alternative methods, and there is a fair amount of confusion in relation to them. There are many different methods and very little evidence of their efficiency. Even the "official" therapy given by physiotherapists fails to demonstrate good effects in scientific studies, probably because of the ineffectiveness of standard medical treatment that patients do not even visit their doctors but instead go directly to a medically unqualified acupuncturist or a chiropractor. This choice has its downsides, because these professionals often do not have sufficient knowledge of medicine, and they try things they should not; in this manner they may even harm the patient. In my opinion, it would be good practice to always start by conducting a medical exam in order to avoid problems.

This is a list of some existing methods, just to give an idea of the variety: acupuncture, moxibustion, several schools of chiropractice, osteopathy, manipulation and mobilization, stretching techniques, various massage techniques as the Swedish massage, transverse friction (Cyriax), ischemic compression, myofascial release, soft tissue mobilization, lymphatic massage, connective tissue massage, sports massage, Rolfing, Alexander technique, oscillation, Russian massage, reflexology, acupressure, shiatsu, and many others. There is a good variety in apparatus, too. Here are some of the most traditional: infrared (heat), ultrasound, electrical stimulation, laser, and magnetic fields.

Each therapy has its followers and works in some cases, but I get many patients who have already visited several therapists without having cured their problems. I think that the education in diagnostic skills of the different therapists is very poor, and that they should learn several treatment techniques in order to have more complete treatments and better results.

It seems to be nonsense to me when a therapist says that in order to find out if the technique helps, it requires at least ten to fifteen sessions. If any technique is effective, you can usually notice at least some improvement after one to five sessions. If not, you have to question either the technique or the skills and find another solution. Promoting many treatments without substantial effect sounds more like a money-spinning business than therapy.

Having personally tested and partially used a variety of methods and devices, my current form of treatment and my combination of treatment methods has crystallized in the combination, which I explain in this book. Successful treatment is based on a good diagnosis and localization of the affected tissues. In myofascial pain, the muscles and tendons are contracted, lack irrigation, and are hardened. The important thing is to have it crystal clear what you intend to treat. The goal of the treatment is to normalize the metabolism, elasticity, and function of the affected tissue, so as to restore mobility and to correct the causes of pain in order to prevent relapses. Good teamwork between the doctor and the therapist is important. The most effective treatment is achieved by focusing the treatment to the sites of maximal pain, called tender points or trigger points.

Treatment with oral anti-inflammatories and analgesics is rarely curative. The symptoms are perhaps relieved while taking the medication, and many patients take medicines for months or even years against pain. Usually if they stop, the pain is there as much as before taking any medication. These drugs are not harmless and have many serious side effects. In order to cure the tissues, they must be treated with methods that also use manual treatments—the so-called deactivation of the painful points.

I have achieved the best results in treatment with the following combination of techniques.

1. Infiltrations or dry needling

2. Any device that facilitates relaxation and circulation

3. Appropriate massage technique

4. Stretching and mobilisation

5. Correct the causes by the application of ergonomics, posture correction, etc.

1. Infiltration

The first component of the treatment is infiltration; a second option is the technique called dry needling. Infiltration has at least four therapeutic effects.

1. Local circulation increases

2. The liquid rinses the tissues and helps to remove accumulated metabolites

3. It has a muscle relaxing effect

4. It reduces pain in order to be able to manipulate the tissues more effectively

By adding steroids, we also achieve a anti-inflammatory effect.

When there is no inflammation, for the infiltrations I use a local anaesthetic of 0.2-0.5 per cent lidocaine (Seyffarth). I do not recommend infiltrations with sterile water; they do not make the results better and are really painful. In one session, I use 20-30 ml of this liquid, injecting 1-3 ml per location. In very sensitive points, I use 1 per cent lidocaine. As a rule, it can be dangerous to anesthetize excessively. The patient will feel much less, and it is easier to overdo the manual treatment, where pain serves as a guide for the graduation of the applied pressure.

The infiltrations are made at the areas of maximum pain, and they are found by using palpation; you also feel a different resistance of the different tissues when you push the needle in, so this feeling can orientate you. Injections of a stronger anaesthetic help to diagnose and find the tissues that are causing the pain; it is called diagnostic local anaesthesia and is a very useful tool (see chapter seven).

In my experience, the infiltrations are more effective than puncture with acupuncture needles, or treatment with any apparatus. I have been able to make comparisons during many years of practicing this technique. With people who are terrified of needles (especially children), I use a TNS-type apparatus or a laser. The effect is individual; some respond better to TNS and others to the laser. There are a large variety of treatment devices, from ultrasound to electromagnets. They all have some positive effects but are not as effective as the infiltrations. Carrying out the treatment without infiltration needs many more sessions; the time and the cost of treatments will then increase.

The most potent method to treat inflammation is currently corticosteroid infiltration. Yet it seems premature to assess the results using botulin toxin. All oral medication or injected intramuscular or intravenous medicines are distributed to almost all areas of the body equally; only a small part reaches the affected area. By infiltrating, the maximum effect is achieved at the infiltrated affected areas and with a minimal amount of medication!

The highly concentrated and strong corticosteroids have the danger of tissue atrophy! This can be avoided by diluting with physiologic saline solution. In relatively short treatments involving infiltrating steroids once or twice a week, there are barely any problems. The fear of steroids that many people and even doctors have is totally irrelevant! The oral or local anti-inflammatory painkillers have their utility when combined with infiltrations in some cases, especially when the patient has severe, continuous ache.

2. Treatment with Different Devices

The devices that reduce pain, increase circulation, help metabolism, and relax muscles are of great help, although they are not entirely necessary. I personally use one of these three: an infrared laser, an electrical transcutaneous acupuncture device, or an electromagnetic device to provide deep heat

3. Massages

Manual therapy (massage) of the tissues is an essential component in the treatment. Infiltration as a sole treatment, or using different apparatus or manipulation (chiropractic) methods alone, is not sufficient to be effective pain treatment. In my personal experience, the most effective way to deactivate trigger points is the combination of injections, deep massage techniques, and manipulations. The manual treatment aims to normalize the tissue metabolism, function, and elasticity. The pain disappears, and the treatment dissolves the contractures.

Massage warms and relaxes tissues by increasing metabolism. It increases circulation and drives out irritating metabolites, thereby decreasing the pain. This is a curative treatment.

It is important that the therapist, with his hands, can find the points and feel the contractures and work consciously to deactivate them. The ability of the therapist is more important than the name of the technique he uses. You have to direct the force of the massage so that the muscle (tissue) to be treated is between the therapist's hand and a firm surface such as a bone, or take the muscle between the fingers. If the massage does not hurt a little, it is not effective!

The treatment zone must be limited. For example, have a session for the neck and shoulders, and another session for the lower back or buttocks. If we try to treat too many big areas, such as doing a full-body massage in one hour, no place will receive sufficient treatment, and the results are poor or non-existent.

The tissues need time to warm up and to gradually accept more pressure. At the start there is added tenderness and pain. When heated, the tissues tolerate stronger pressure in order to gradually be able to reach deeper layers. Usually the pain begins to fade after ten to twenty minutes of massage, and the muscle begins to feel softer. If we start with excessive pressure, it hurts too much, and we can easily create bruising and frighten the patient so that he might never be back. The tolerance of each patient is highly individual and must be respected. A too-short massage never reaches the deeper layers, and a too-long or too-hard massage causes unnecessary pain and soreness many days after the treatment.

This is how I usually divide the time of a session that lasts fifty to sixty minutes (for a limited area). I use about ten to twenty minutes to locate the problems and infiltrate the points of maximal soreness, and another five to ten minutes to apply some of my apparatus. The massage takes twenty to thirty minutes. The remaining time is for stretching, manipulation, and instructions.

Different massage techniques are used according to each individual case. It's good to know a variety of techniques in order to be able choose and combine. The techniques can be classified by their purpose, such as the lymph drainage massage that serves to remove oedemas. There is another massage for the venous return. The so-called connective tissue massage treats cellulitis and hardened subcutaneous areas with poor metabolism and scar tissue, as often happens with the legs that have had varicose ulcers or when the lymphatic glands have been removed. The deep muscle massage relaxes the muscles, deactivates the trigger points, removes the contractures, and returns the original elasticity to the muscle. Finally, there are techniques to treat ligaments, tendons, and joint capsules. You must always keep in mind the goal: what do you intend to achieve with your treatment?

I'm going to give a few of examples of the choice of techniques for different cases.

1. Treatment of trigger points and muscle spasms in the buttock and lateral thigh (sciatica). I start with a warming-up technique. I use the Furter technique, which

is done using oil and then gliding the knuckles in quick movements in the direction of the muscle fibres with very little pressure, especially in the thigh area. It is usually very painful, and you have to start very lightly. Another more pleasant possibility is to use rubbing strokes with the palm of the hand, using oil. When the tissue is heated, I concentrate the massage to the painful areas, kneading deeper and varying cross-sectional or longitudinal or oblique stokes, or using a circular motion, until the tension and the hardness has disappeared. This usually requires a few sessions.

2. A swollen arm after lymph node dissection and radiation therapy (breast cancer). The oedema in these cases is usually of very hard consistency. For permanent results, the lymphatic massage technique is not sufficient. The treatment must also encourage the deeper return circulation. and there is a need of venous return and connective tissue massage techniques.

    For connective tissue massage, I do not use the original technique, which is extremely painful. The same effect is achieved with the pinching technique. The pinching can be easily adjusted so that the treatment is better tolerated. It is entirely possible to cure such cases, but it often requires many (ten to fifteen) sessions.

3. Calf pain, oedematous calf with ulcers or scars after thrombophlebitis or cellulitis. The skin has often brown pigmentation as a sign of poor venous circulation and poor tissue metabolism. In these cases, the infiltration with local anaesthetic is extremely important because the treatment causes considerable pain. The liquid forced into the hard and scarred tissue is loosening the tissue and creating space for the natural fluids that will flow better and begin to nurture and heal the tissue. Combine the circulatory massage with the connective tissue massage.

4. Tendons, joint capsules, and fascia. The knee has usually many sore points in the tendons, joint capsule, retinacula, and the bursa. I mostly use infiltration with corticosteroids—for example, 4 mg of dexamethasone diluted to 5-10 cc, infiltrating 0.5-2.0 cc at each point. Sometimes to find the locations, I use a round-tipped stick because the finger is too big to localize the points with precision.

Tendon injuries also require massage (and rest) for the healing and restoration of the metabolism. I often use a technique of fast friction with oil (by Dr Furter) with a round-headed stick or my knuckles. As an alternative and less painful technique, I use deep transverse massage with the fingers. The treatment of the ankle and the wrist are very similar.

Remember that when there is pain in a tendon, the corresponding muscle may be affected and contractured, and in order to heal the tendon, you must also heal the muscle. If we leave the muscle tense and strained, the tendon cannot improve.

4. Mobilization

After the massage and when the muscles are warmed up, I proceed to the joint mobilization and stretching of muscles and tendons that restrict the movements. The slow stretch mobilizations are safer than chiropractic techniques and are almost always sufficient. Most of the time the stretching done at the therapy sessions is not enough. Tissues need daily stretching to acquire their original length, and you must instruct the patients how to stretch at home.

Chiropractic manipulations are rarely necessary, and you should be very careful with these techniques. Deaths have occurred after the manipulation of the cervical spine, and manipulation of the lumbar spine may lead to emergency surgery if the prolapsed disc moves and increases the compression on the sciatic nerve.

5. Ergonomics and Relapse Prevention

An important part of treatment is to try to correct the causes of the complaints so that problems do not come back and the same mistakes are not repeated. You have to correct poor postures and teach the correct pedestation, as well as how to walk and sit correctly, and how to work in ergonomically correct postures without unnecessary tension. Teaching techniques of correct lifting are important. Instruct how to avoid overloading muscles with monotonous work, especially when the body is not used and trained to it.

Some patients need relaxation exercises for their stress and nervous tension, which also causes muscle tension; this is often unconscious. Common areas for nervous tension are the shoulders, the back, or the masticators. There are many anti-stress methods. One of the easiest to learn is a self-hypnosis and relaxation practice at home with the help of a recording, or practicing some easy meditation techniques. For heavy localized tensions, there are some simple biofeedback methods that help to get rid of the tensing habits.

In other cases there is need to strengthen certain muscles so that their tolerance increases. In general people need to be taught how to use the body correctly. Let us take a very common example. The tension in the neck with a possible headache is often caused by poor posture. When seated, we lean back to sink down, and as a consequence the head is placed too forward. At times we place our head even more forwards to see the computer screen or the book we read. At this posture the muscles have to continually support the weight of the head, and it creates a muscle overload so that gradually the muscles start to hurt.

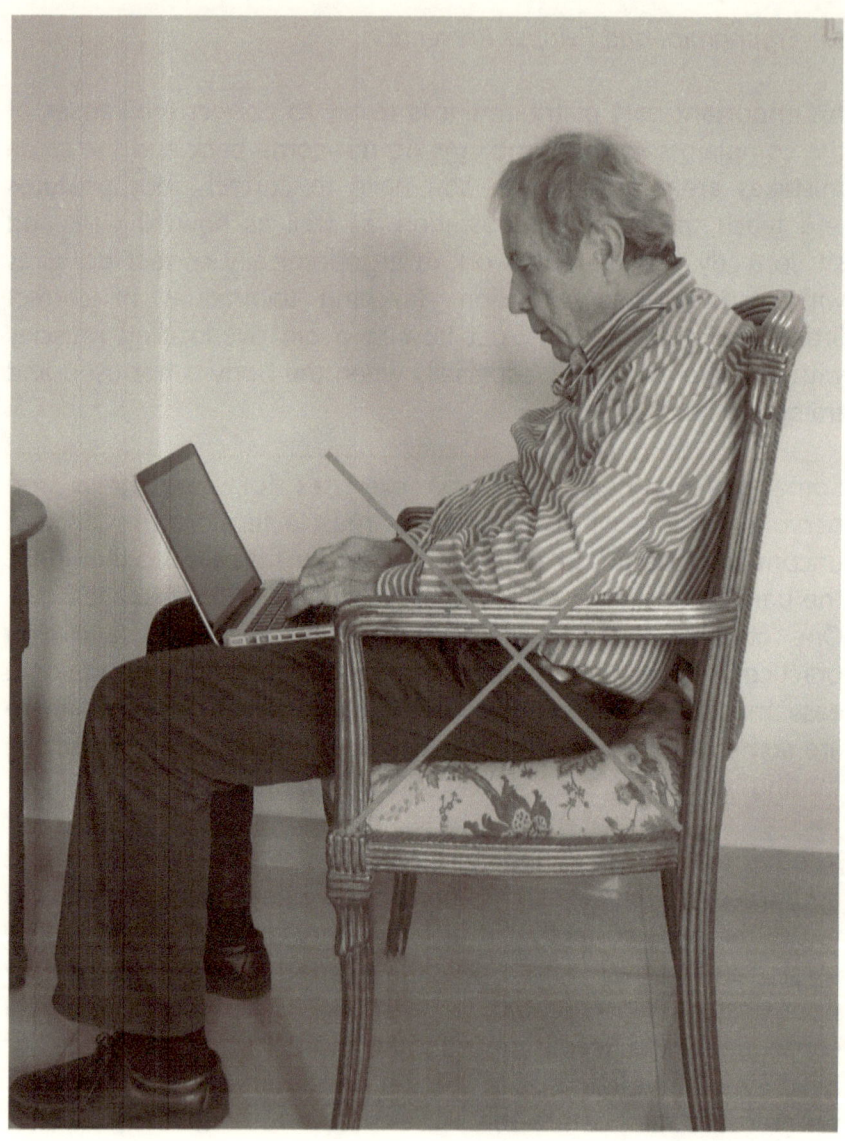

The worst thing for the muscles is continuous tension, called static muscle work, even with a minimal load. The prolonged contraction inhibits circulation and metabolism. Metabolites accumulate and gradually begin to irritate the pain nerve endings.

9. THE HEAD

Pain in the head may have a myofascial origin, but first we must rule out other diseases and be sure there are not any serious illnesses behind the symptoms. The head muscles can be overstrained and cause pain. Furthermore, the muscles of the neck and shoulders can radiate pain to the head and even trigger headaches or trap nerves.

The causes are often related to stress and nervous tension, which makes us tense various muscles in the head area. A common nervous habit is to clench the teeth, often during sleep. This habit (often unconscious) activates trigger points in the masticator muscles such as the temporalis muscle (myofascial pain can be confused with temporal arteritis!), the masseter muscle, and sometimes the pterygoid muscle. This can cause problems in the temporo-mandibular joint and the teeth. The image shows common location of trigger points in this area.

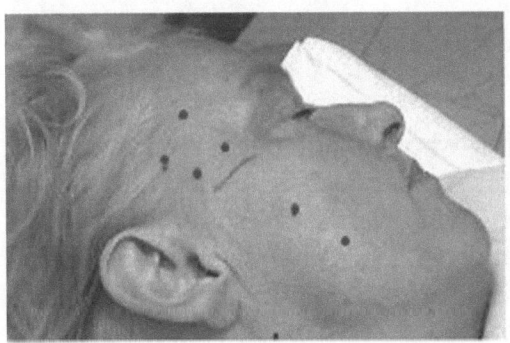 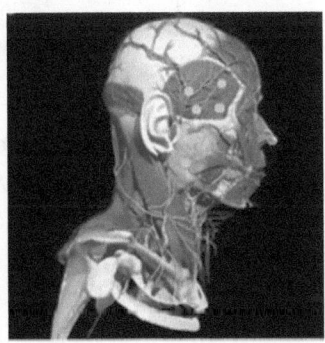

Picture: "3D univadis Anatomiamalli",
Copyright © Primal Pictures Ltd.

Another major cause of headaches is the neck muscles, which reflect the pain to the head. Patients with headache should be checked for painful points of the neck and the shoulders. This chapter includes the muscles of the skull base. (The neck has its own chapter.)

There are several layers of muscles at the base of the skull, and all of them can develop trigger points. The greater occipital nerve goes through the semispinalis capitis and trapezius muscles. When these are tense and swollen, the nerve can be trapped and inflamed. The occipital pain points often send radiation to the eye area. Muscle tension may be a result of tension and stress of psychological origin, or of poor posture and other bad habits. Poor posture of the neck, especially the pre-emption of the head, is very common (see photos below).

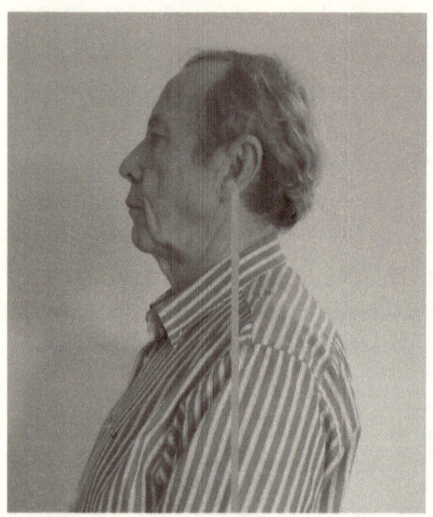 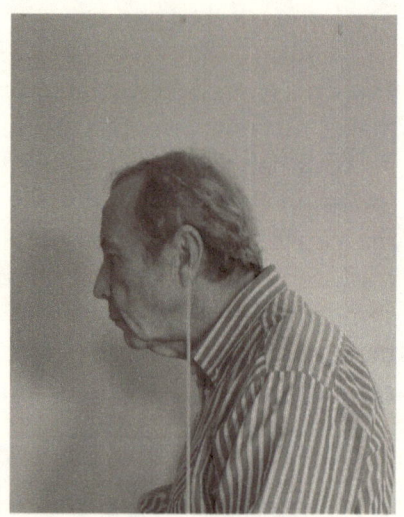

There are very few patients who do not need a correction of their posture and their work ergonomics. Examples of common causes are all sedentary jobs that give rise to tension in the neck: crafts, using a computer, and reading. Other causes could be an inadequate pillow or the habit of reading in bed and holding the book in an awkward position.

During a clinical examination of headache, it is important that the patients are being differentiated from intracranial diseases and other not muscular diseases. A basic blood test and possible imaging studies to exclude other, more serious diseases is recommended.

In this area there are many different possible causes of pain, such as infections of the teeth or sinuses, swollen temporal arteries, or trigeminal neuralgias. Intracranial causes are migraine headaches, certain infections, and tumours. We must look for signs of neurological disorders, palpate the different glands, feel and listen to the arteries, examine the mobility of the neck, and palpate the areas where there may be trigger points.

Myofascial Treatment

Without correcting the posture and bad habits, the results of myofascial treatments are often poor or short lived. Whenever we find painful trigger points, we have to think of the possible causes of overstrain in those muscles and try to correct the causes! The habit of unconsciously tensing the muscles is a barrier to achieving positive results. Patients must learn to relax. There are several methods to achieve relaxation, from methods of biofeedback and meditation to yoga and relaxation techniques. In order to correct the posture of the head, there is a very simple biofeedback method: place a ribbon in the way the picture shows.

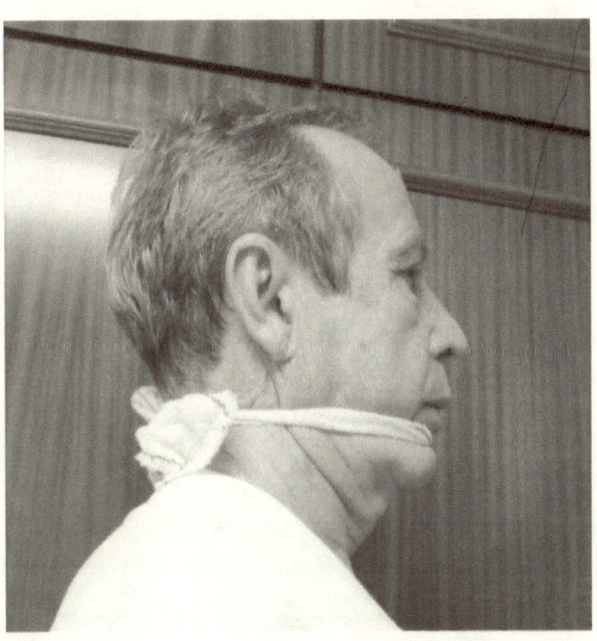

It will inhibit the pre-emption of the head. Remember that the correction of the posture starts from below, from the correct position of the back.

Bruxism requires that the dentist manufacture a device known as a bite bar, which is kept in the mouth at nights. The patient should also practice general relaxation techniques. One of the most effective and easy to learn is self-hypnosis.

Stress and poor posture are not easily corrected and need time, but these steps are necessary to prevent relapse. The painful points are infiltrated and massaged until cured. The muscles of the neck and jaw need stretching exercises (see chapter ten). The companion video demonstrates the technique of treating the most common areas. You also have to consider the need of treating the neck and shoulders in connection with head problems.

10. THE NECK

The neck is a vital part of the body and is an area in which many people have problems. Neck pain can radiate upwards and cause headaches and pain in the ear, or it can radiate down and cause pain in the shoulders and arms. Neck problems may be related to dizziness and vertigo. Throat pain when swallowing may also have myofascial origin in the small muscles of this area (the treatment is called voice massage). Again, the osteoarthritis is too often blamed for the pain. Remember that osteoarthritis itself does not cause any significant pain—the pains are almost always caused by the soft parts that can be treated and almost always cured, or at least considerably eased.

Causes and Activation Mechanisms

A stressful and sedentary lifestyle is probably the major cause of painful conditions in the neck. Our neck is the main place to accumulate stress and tension, and it even has a name: the tension neck syndrome. With stress and anxiety, we often tend to tense the muscles of the neck and shoulders, gradually activating trigger points. Another common cause is poor posture and unhealthy working positions. Wrong posture affects the neck column; the muscles are continuously tense, and they become overworked and painful.

The most common posture is the pre-emption of the head. (See photo in the previous chapter). This pre-emption is caused when we let our back sink into a relaxed position and it is curved forward. Furthermore, poor posture while standing or walking causes the dislocation of the neck and head of its natural balanced position.

When the point of gravity of the head is in front of the vertebral column, muscle work is needed to keep the head in position, and consequently the muscles become overworked. The muscular memory of the position is gradually programmed to accept the bad posture as normal and natural, and what would be the correct posture would feel weird. This makes the correction of postures difficult. A new programming of the muscle memory is needed, and it requires a substantial effort to reprogram the muscles to adapt correct posture again.

Other causes of muscular overload are habits such as supporting the phone between the shoulder and the ear, or having the head turned to one side when the TV is not in front of you, or in a classroom always being seated in the same side. When we read books and do crafts, we have the book, the screen, or the handiwork placed so that we have to tilt our head forward for a considerable time, and thus we overwork the muscles of the neck.

After some time, the poor posture and tensions increases stiffness and limitation of movement, and it accelerates the formation of osteoarthritis. The most limiting for the neck rotation are the contractures in the scalene muscles; the limitation in flexion extension usually develops in a much later stage. Contractures develop by not stretching the neck enough and by not using the whole movement range.

The neck can be injured in falls and car accidents (whiplash). I have had many patients with chronic pain after whiplash accidents, without any injury to be seen on radiographs or MRI. According to a German study, it is recommended to perform an MRI in the acute phase. The soft-tissue injuries show clearer while there is still the acute inflammatory reaction. This study is important because the early MRI can provide concrete evidence to insurance companies and other officials; later, the signs disappear. Trauma might well increase the rate of progression of osteoarthritis, although this is difficult to prove. The post-traumatic pain is most often caused by soft tissues, which are the muscles and the ligaments, and they can improve with this treatment.

Prolapsed cervical discs with trapped nerve roots are also quite common. They can be produced by lifting heavy weights or even by extreme coughing. Sometimes the differential diagnosis between muscle pain and radiculitis caused by a prolapsed disc can be difficult. Remember that when there is a doubt, you can practice a gentle longitudinal traction of the cervical spine; in the case of a prolapse, pain tends to decrease. Traction is also the treatment choice in these cases. There are other types of nervous entrapments, such as the anterior scalenus syndrome (the Adson test), the claviculo-costal syndrome, and the impingement of the occipital nerves.

As in many other places, when there is pain in the neck, one starts to tense the muscles as a form of protection, thus causing a vicious circle where this tension causes even more pain.

The Examination

First observe the position of the patient standing and sitting. Palpate muscles to find points of pain and tension. Examine the movements and whether they are painful or limited. Examine the rotation, flexion-extension, and lateral flexion. Dorsiflexion combined with rotation reduces the nerve foramina of the side of rotation and decreases the space of the nerve passage. I mentioned earlier that traction helps to differentiate between the trapped nerve pain and the myofascial pain. (Patients with osteoporosis and rheumatoid arthritis must be examined and treated very gently, due to the fragility of their vertebrae and ligaments.) The photographs have marked the most common myofascial pain points in this area.

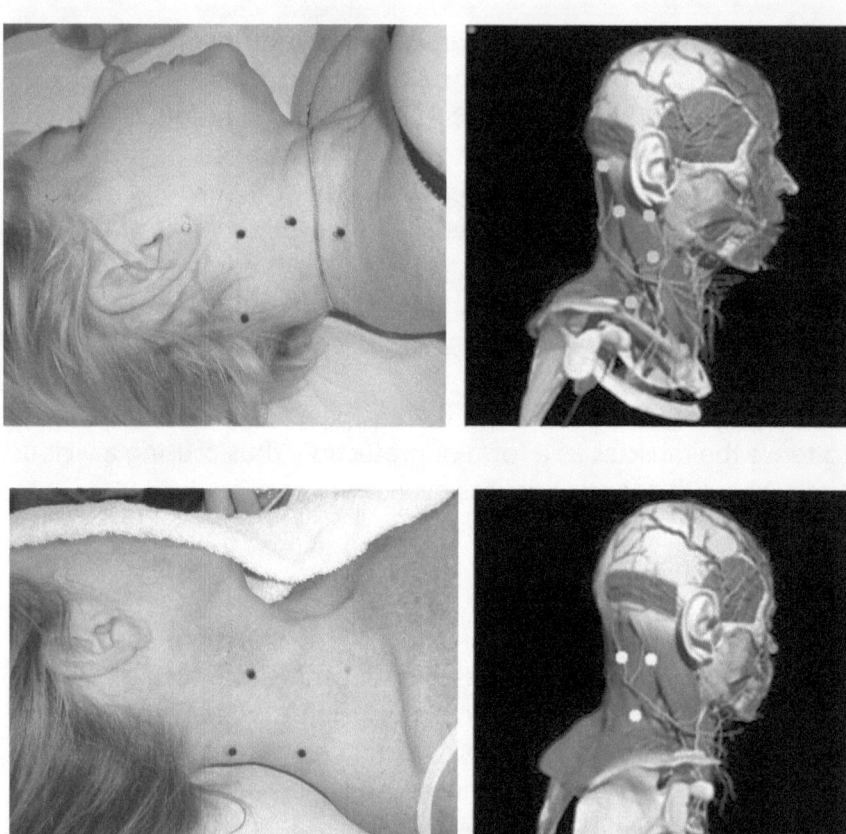

Univadis/3D Anatomiamalli, Copyright © Primal Pictures Ltd

For the differential diagnosis, it may be necessary to have blood tests and X-rays or MRI scans.

The Treatment

Therapists can be reluctant to treat the side of the neck because of the proximity to the large vessels and nerves. However, the lateral muscles are very important in the treatment, especially the scalenus muscles, the sternocleidomastoid, and the levator scapulae muscles. These muscles are very often contracted and have painful trigger points. The shortening of these muscles is the main cause of reduced neck mobility. These muscles can be treated when one well knows anatomy. The treatment consists of infiltrating or dry needling the points of maximal pain, then treating with some apparatus to heat and relax the muscles. Massage and stretching re-establish the metabolism and muscle function.

The sides of the neck are massaged in the face-up position by turning the head slightly to the side. The back part is done in a face-down position on a table with a hole for the face, or with a special support device (picture) and the patient sitting.

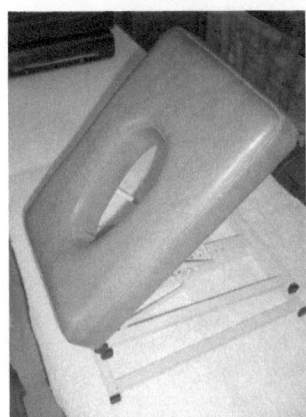 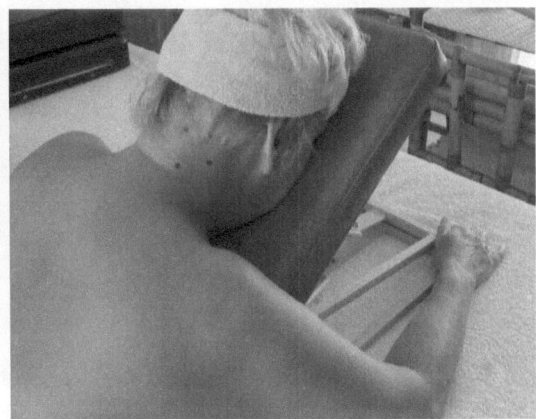

It is vital to stretch the lateral muscles (Image) and the patient has to do the stretching at home **daily**. It's also beneficial to stretch the posterior neck muscles. Stretching should be smooth without jerks, stretching slowly to the point where it starts to hurt and maintain for 15-20 seconds.

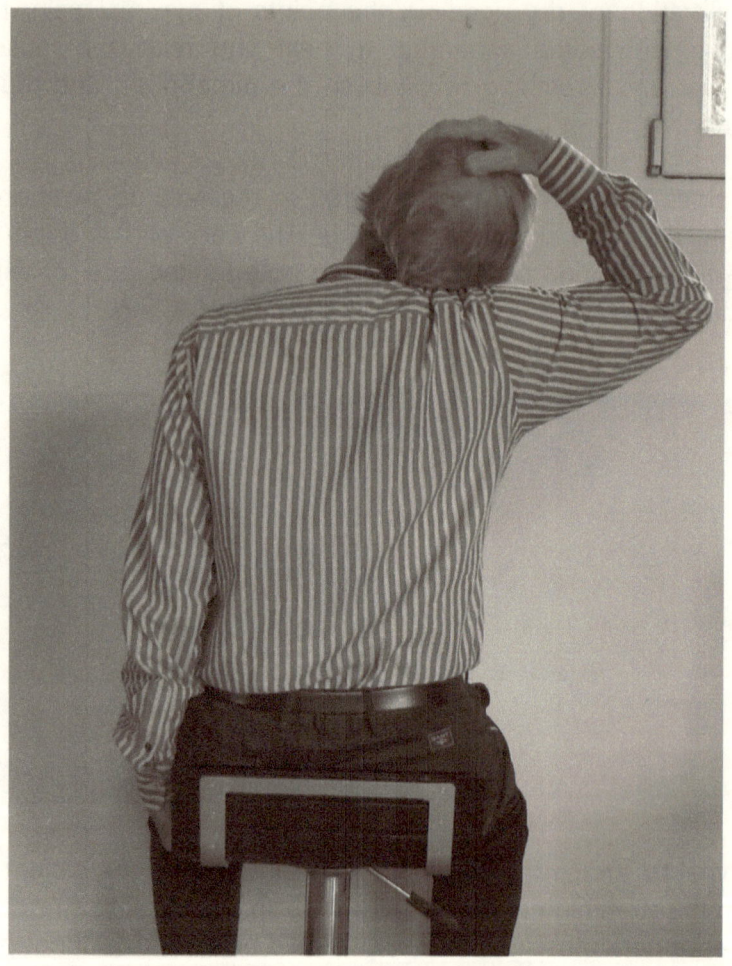

Gradually, with days and weeks of daily stretching, the muscles regain their length. Often it is also advisable to do longitudinal tractions. Chiropractic manipulations are in most cases unnecessary (and are not totally safe) because the relaxation, stretching, and mobilization of muscles and tendons is sufficient to regain the mobility.

Ergonomics and Posture

Of equal importance as the treatment of the muscles is the correction of the posture and habits. Changing old habits is not easy, but is the only way to prevent relapses. The patient has to start continuous self control until he has created a new habit with the correct posture and use of his muscles. To help with this complex task, there are some quite simple biofeedback methods; there are even sophisticated electronic biofeedback devices, but these are usually very expensive.

Against pre-emption of the head, one uses a ribbon, which is tied around the neck and around the chin. The loop has to be inelastic and tense so that it does not allow the forward movement of the head and continually reminds the patient of the correct position, but it still allows flexion-extension and rotation. The balance of the head is achieved only if the back also has the correct posture, as in the following pictures.

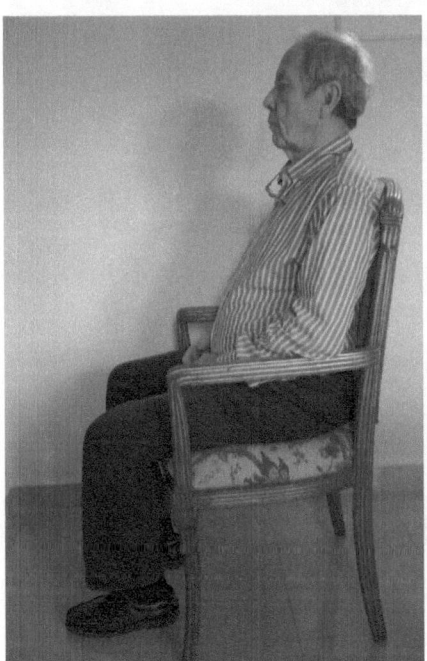 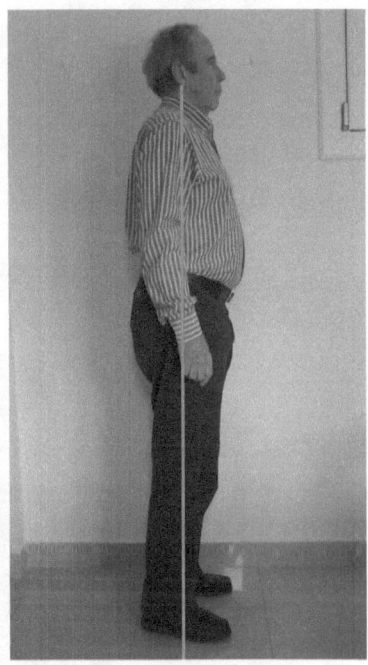

The position must be corrected starting from the knees, which must not be hyperextended but should be loose. One must have the correct pelvic tilt, and the back straight should be but relaxed; the shoulders should be relaxed as well.

Against tension and the wrong habit of raising the shoulders, there is another easy biofeedback method. Use an adhesive, no-elastic bandage (sports tape), which is glued to the skin like a suspender when the patient holds his shoulders down. Every time he forgets and raises the shoulders, he feels a tug in his skin.

We must review the ergonomics and postures of the daily tasks performed by each patient, and we must especially pay attention to reduce static muscle work.

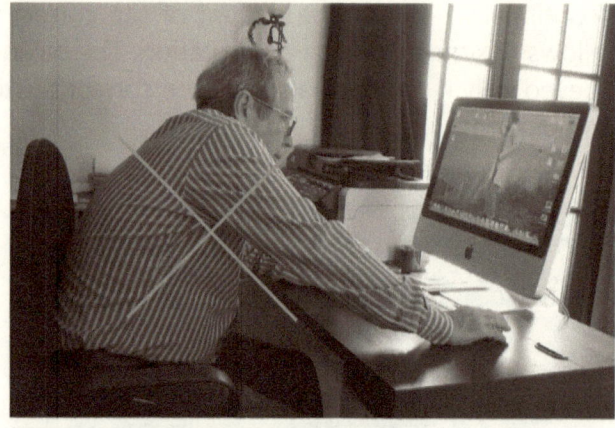

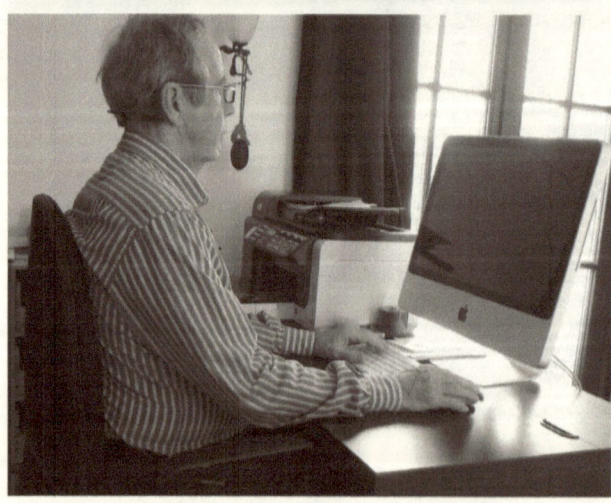

The ergonomically correct position to work with your computer.

11. THE SHOULDER

The shoulder joint is the most complicated part of the body, especially because it easily creates a vicious circle where pain causes tension, and the tension blocks the movements and causes an erroneous movement pattern that continues to irritate the tissues. The fact that the patient tenses up the shoulder (involuntary and unconscious, because of the pain) narrows the space of the supraspinatus tendon and the rotator cuff. In each movement there is increased friction to the tendons and the joint capsule; this maintains the irritation and inflammation as well as the pain. The pain furthermore causes limited motion, and within a few weeks and months, the muscles and tendons shrink, causing a progressive reduction in the movement range. The result is a frozen shoulder.

Because of the facts above, it is very important to treat the different stages of this condition in a particular order, and to instruct the patient thoroughly in the exercises and the allowed movements, regarding how to do everything without tension and with the right movement pattern.

The Causes

Here is a list of the common causes of shoulder pain.

1. Acute or Chronic Overload: Examples of an acute overload would be to lift heavy things without having the practice or training for it—for example, carrying heavy suitcases or lifting furniture. Another example is to overload the shoulder with repetitive movements, such as cleaning windows, sweeping, painting walls, and hairdressing. Chronic overload takes longer time to produce pain, maybe even years. As examples I could mention monotonous work movements: those of a painter, a carpenter, or a masseuse. Another common cause is posture causing prolonged tension, such as holding books or newspapers in

arms, knitting, or using the computer mouse in awkward and tense postures. Even if the force used in these cases is not extensive, this prolonged static tension in the muscles can block the circulation. The oxygen and the nutrients cannot enter, and the metabolites cannot leave the muscle and the accumulation slowly blocks the function and activates the trigger points.

2. Trauma: Injuries cause an inflammation reaction to the tissues (muscle, tendon, joint capsule, and nerve), with signs of local swelling, pain, and sometimes heat. In cases with fractures or ruptures of tendons, it is important to evaluate whether the treatment should be surgical or conservative. Especially in the shoulder, the rapid and effective treatment of the pain and inflammation with early mobilization, and teaching the patient the right movements (see the treatment part), is of vital importance to avoid prolonged painful conditions and the reduction of the movement range, so that the movement range does not have time to be significantly reduced.

3. Neuropathic Pain: Pain caused by a trapped nerve in this area can be confusing and sometimes difficult to distinguish from myofascial pain, and both may even exist simultaneously. The nerve entrapment has a completely different treatment procedure.

4. Pain caused by inflammatory diseases. such as poly myalgia rheumatica, rheumatoid arthritis. and other forms of arthritis must also be treated medically.

5. Other painful diseases such as fibromyalgia, which in 60 per cent of cases also has active myofascial trigger points. The deactivation of the myofascial trigger points gives at least a partial relief, even in these patients.

How to Examine Patients with Shoulder Pain

A good clinical history and a thorough examination of the area are important to diagnose a patient correctly. History often already reveals the cause of the pain. In cases which involve trauma, you should take X-rays. When there are signs of a ruptured tendon, ultrasound or an MRI are indicated. To rule out inflammatory or rheumatic diseases, sedimentation rate and CRP are minimally required.

The first thing is to ask the patient to indicate the painful sites and to show the painful and restricted movements. You cannot do a good examination without asking the patient to undress. The visual inspection is to notice any abnormality in colour, contour, position, or atrophy. Then with a light touch, you notice changes in temperature. You examine the circulation and the neurological status. The movements are examined first with passive movements, internal and external rotation, and lifting the arm. The next step is to examine the active movements and their limitations. It is important to observe whether the humero-claviculo-scapular movement pattern is correct; when the supraspinatus tendon has a total rupture, lateral arm abduction is not possible.

Carefully palpate and locate the spots of maximum pain for the treatment. Apart from the pain points of the shoulder, the cervical area should be palpated: the trapezius muscle, the scapular zone, the pectoral muscles, and even the axilla, because all influence in the function and pain of the shoulder. Arthrosis and the inflammation of the claviculo-scapular joint cause similar symptoms as supraspinatus tendinitis.

It is sometimes difficult to distinguish between myofascial pain and neuropathic pain (cervical impingement). The rotation and lateral flexion test of the neck towards the affected shoulder discovers the cervical prolapse. If there is pain when carrying out this test on the opposite side, it might be sign of scalenus syndrome. You can also find prolapsed discs by practicing a longitudinal traction to the cervical spine. The pain is alleviated for the duration of traction. By anesthetizing painful points one by one, we can find the tissue that is causing the pain. In the photographs you can see the most common locations of the painful points.

This man is suffering from playing golf.

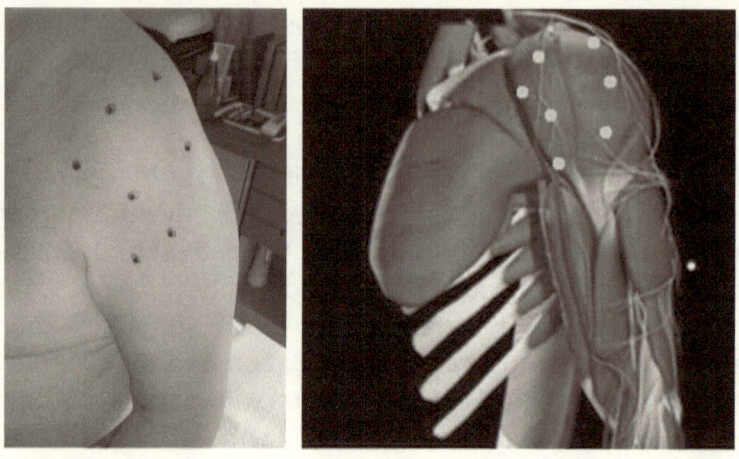

This shoulder hurts after a fall and a jerk.

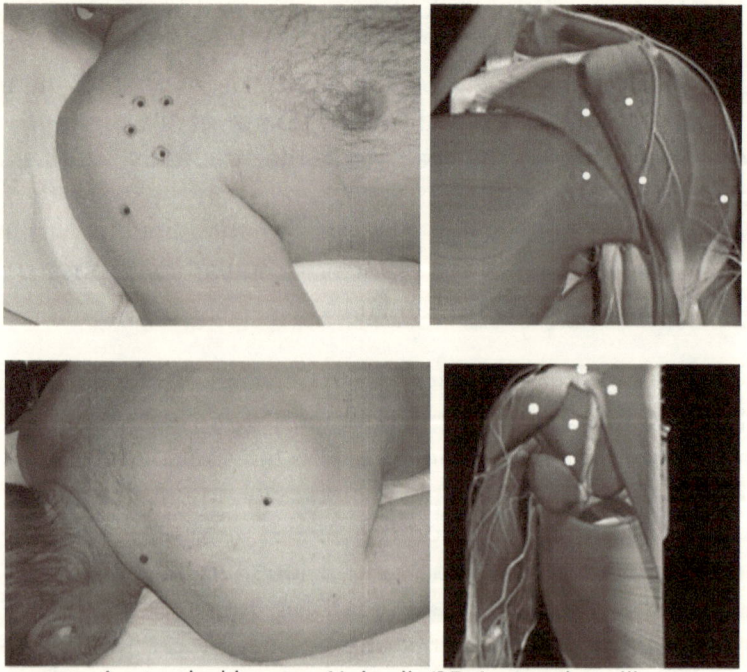

Anatomical images: Univadis/3D Anatomiamalli,
Copyright © Primal Pictures Ltd.

She felt deep pain in the shoulder blade area.

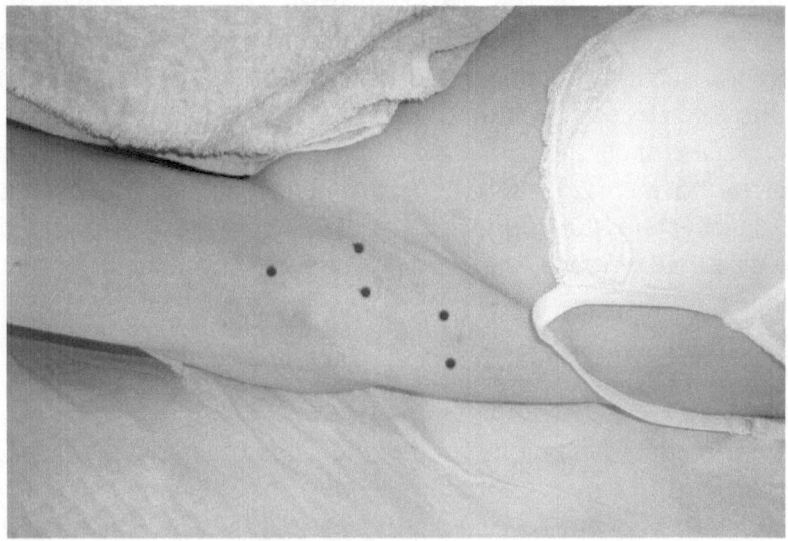

In this example, the overload was caused by painting six months ago. The external rotation was reduced by the shrinking of the pectoral muscles. Also, the supraspinatus tendon was swollen, and arm elevation was painful.

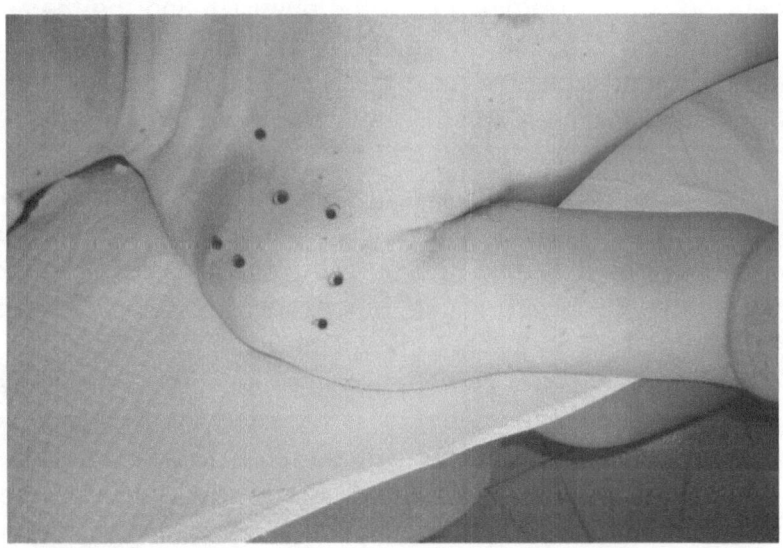

Different Diagnostics Labels Given to Patients with Myofascial Pain

The following diagnoses are used: frozen shoulder, periarthritis, bursitis, tendinitis, golfer's shoulder, prolonged post-traumatic pain (sprains, fractures), sprains, and partial ruptures of the ligaments or the rotator cuff. In all these painful conditions, the treatment is similar. First of all, the pain and the inflammation are treated (heavy exercise to increase strength and mobility are contraindicated!) by deactivating the trigger points. After that we can begin the exercises to increase the mobility and getting the ergonomics right.

The Treatment

The shoulder is unique regarding treatment, as I already mentioned. The greatest danger is that the movements become very restricted—the so-called frozen shoulder. The other danger is that the pain and limited movement can easily become chronic. For this reason we must begin to mobilize quickly, but here are some tricks for how to do it correctly.

Inadequate mobilization exercises, at the wrong time, often only aggravate the problem. Treatment must be carried out in a specific order, and so the coordination of the physician and the therapist is vital! When the pain is severe and the ache makes sleep difficult or impossible, the main thing is to treat the pain and the inflammation as quickly and efficiently as possible.

The most effective method, in my experience, is totally immobilize the shoulder in a sling, giving it absolute rest. Then infiltrate the painful and inflamed tissues with corticosteroid and local anaesthetic. I use the mixture of one per cent lidocaine with 4mg dexamethasone a total amount of 5cc and infiltrate points of greatest pain (2 to 5 points in one session). This usually gives very good results. The infiltration is repeated the next day, and if needed again after two or three days. (The intra-articular corticosteroid injection is usually not as effective.) Added to these measures, I prescribe a potent oral anti-inflammatory medication and a muscle relaxant if needed. The important thing is to cure the constant pain as soon as possible; usually it takes one to three days.

After this begins phase two of the treatment. The constant pain is now gone, but the shoulder still hurts in certain movements.

At this stage we must begin the mobilization and simultaneously continue the pain treatment. The first exercises must be carried out with totally relaxed muscles and with passive movements. The patient takes his arm out of the sling two to four times a day and does the following exercise:

Use a light weight in your hand (a water bottle of half a litre); the arm hangs at your side. Swing the arm by moving the body (do not use the shoulder muscles) in the sagittal plane and in the frontal plane for a couple of minutes. Then put the arm back to rest in the sling. This passive exercise stimulates circulation in the shoulder and prevents the freezing of the joint. At the same time, the patient is allowed to use the arm in the painless region with gentle movements, like using the arm for eating.

The treatment of the sore spots continues with infiltration and a manual treatment. I gradually increase the amount of liquid in the infiltrations (for example, 10 cc of 0.25-0.5 per cent local anaesthetic) and decrease the amount of corticosteroid. Now I gradually begin to massage the painful areas. At first the massage is very gentle and is carried out for a shorter time, increasing with each session according to the tolerance of the patient. I start with ten to fifteen minutes and gradually increase the time to the normal twenty to thirty minutes. It is beneficial to use ultrasound, laser, or TNS with the manual treatment. The massage can cause discomfort and soreness in the area, which should not last more than two to three days. If the duration is longer or there is significant pain increase, the treatment has been too evasive.

At the same time, I begin to treat the movement restrictions with gradual, passive stretching exercises. I do this at the end of the session, when the tissues are warmed up. The shortened muscles are slowly stretched to the limit when it starts to hurt; hold them out fifteen to twenty seconds, then repeat the stretch three to four times. The most important stretches are the external and internal rotations, and the elevation. (The elbow must be held into the body when rotating.) The patient must do the same exercises at home, three to four times daily, starting softly and gradually increasing the intensity. Before stretching, the muscles are warmed up by a few second static contractions. Stretching should feel slightly painful to be effective but should not increase the pain afterwards. Now, only partial immobilization and rest are necessary; the patient is only allowed to do light things with his arm that do not cause pain.

The treatment sessions are continued every five to seven days with the injections, massage, and stretching until the total inactivation of the painful points. All the medication is reduced gradually as the pain disappears.

It is very important that you verify the patient does the exercises correctly and raises his arm without tensing the shoulder. It's advisable that the patient carries out the arm-lifting exercises in front of a mirror. There must be no shoulder elevation or tension when the arm is lifted. When there has been pain, the tension is instinctive and mostly unconscious (fear of pain). The patient has to relearn the right movement pattern (see the companion video).

Another important part of the treatment, which is done simultaneously in the course of the sessions, is to try to find the cause of the overload in order to be able to avoid it in the future and correct the ergonomics.

The Different Treatment Positions:

To massage the shoulder trigger points, the position of the shoulder must be changed, depending on the muscle group that is to be treated. The pectorals are best treated in the supine position, with the humerus rotated externally. Regarding the area of the deltoid and supraspinatus, the patient should lie on the opposite side, the arm resting on and parallel to the body. The points of the infraspinatus, teres minor, and teres major muscles are best reached at their distal part, when the patient lies on his side and the humerus is elevated ninety degrees in the sagittal plane. The proximal part of these muscles is caught with the patient lying face down and arms along his side. While the patient lies on his back with his arm raised, we can reach the subscapularis, pectoralis minor, teres major, latissimus dorsi, and toracobraquial muscles.

12. THE ARM AND HAND

The arms have to cope with overloads and tensions. Almost everyone these days owns or accesses a computer. People often work long hours in poor posture, often without supporting the arms and causing tension of the muscles. Other jobs that are highly repetitive, such as painting walls, using a hammer, or trimming hedges, strain the arms a lot if people do not keep the correct posture. Carrying heavy bags on a trip is a common cause of pain in the arms and shoulders. While playing golf and tennis, people can get small injuries (sprains) with the strokes. Musicians often work in unnatural and stressful postures, overloading their muscles and creating painful muscles, tendons, and joints. As always, even if the tension is minor but is sustained for a long period of time, it is not beneficial for the arm and will activate trigger points. For example, holding a book or a newspaper in the arms may cause pain in the long term. Tennis elbow, or lateral epicondylitis, is also a frequent condition. The pain is mostly near the proximal end of the extensor muscles of the fingers and is not only around the epicondyle.

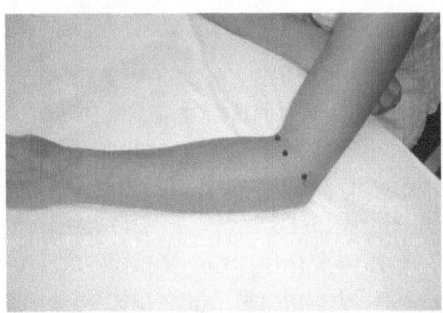 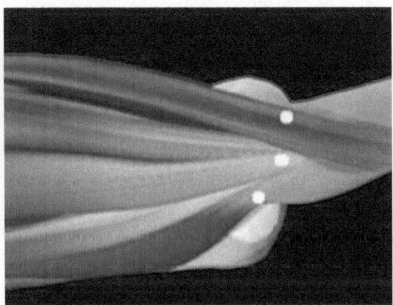

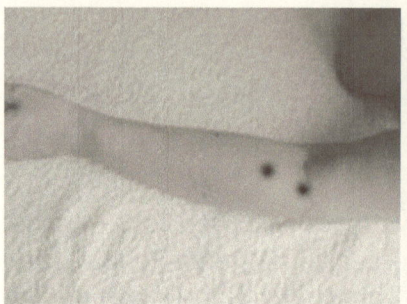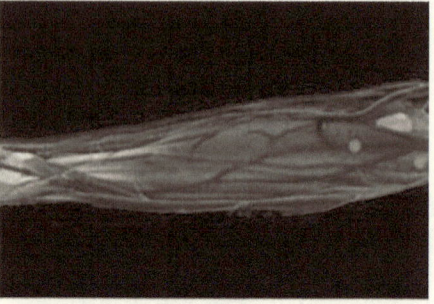

Anatomical images: Univadis/3D Anatomiamalli,
Copyright © Primal Pictures Ltd.

Often a whole muscle group is affected. We must find all the painful points and treat them, because they also affect the tendon. Unfortunately, often the only treatment administered is an injection of corticosteroids into the tendon near the epicondyle—the whole affected muscle has been left without treatment, with a poor result. Furthermore, the flexor side of the underarm can develop painful areas and develop an epicondylitis at the inner epicondyle, called golfer's elbow. In principle, all the arm muscles can be affected (the biceps bacchii, the triceps) and all forearm muscles (the superficial and also the deep layers, such as the supinator muscle).

We must be aware that there are other conditions causing pain in the arm, such as a nerve entrapment in the neck, and then the treatment is different. More rare are the entrapments of distal nerves near the elbow or the cubital tunnel. A fairly common condition is carpal tunnel syndrome. The overuse or poor posture of the wrist, such as when driving a bicycle or sleeping with a flexed wrist, causes an inflammation of the tendons in the narrow channel and begins to compress and irritate the nerve. The result is pain, tingling, and loss of sensation and strength in the hand. The entrapment can be treated successfully, infiltrating a rather large amount of the treatment liquid (with cortisone) around the nerve to create more space and also treating the tense and cramped flexor muscles.

In the hand itself, the adductor and opponent muscles of the thumb receive perhaps the most strain, especially in jobs where one needs to squeeze tools and objects with the fingers. Trigger points of the opponent are usually found in the most proximal part. The hardened muscle cord (trigger point) of the adductors is also proximal, between the first and second metacarpal bones. Massaging them is complicated. The masseuse must take the muscles between his two fingers, or else the muscle "escapes".

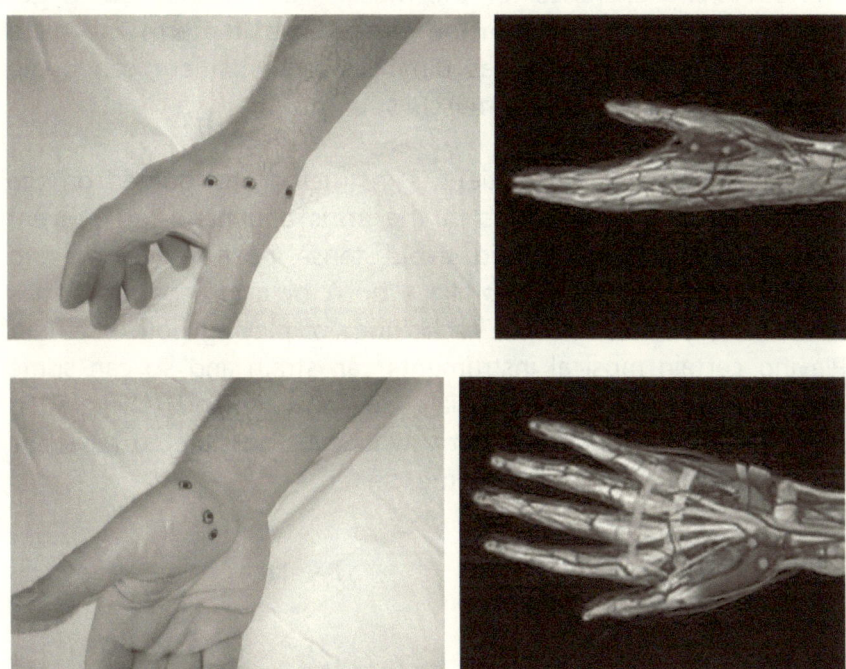

Univadis/3D Anatomiamalli,
Copyright © Primal Pictures Ltd

The frequent pain of osteoarthritis of the fingers and even rheumatoid arthritis of the hand can alleviate much infiltrating small amounts of steroid with lidocaine (0.1-0.2 cc) at the periarticular points of maximal pain. The massage is given to increase the circulation and metabolism. The mobilization of joints is done with a longitudinal traction. The mobilization technique of bending the finger is usually too painful and unnecessary. The patient should make these tractions daily at home. As in other joints, treating the soft tissues around the joint relieves pain and stiffness, but it does not cure arthritis. Osteoarthritis in the fingers has calm periods and periods of inflammation and pain. The cold weather and strains are factors that tend to worsen arthritis.

Treatment in this area follows the same principles of infiltrations and deactivation of the trigger points, softening the hardened muscles and tender points of the tendons and joint capsules. The stretching exercises for the muscles are well suited to get full mobility and to assist in the relaxation of the arm and hand muscles. When the pain has diminished the patient can begin gradual training to increase muscle strength.

It is important that the patient is instructed and guided on the proper use and ergonomics of the arms and hands to prevent relapse. The patient should avoid tense postures or holding certain objects in his hands like a book or a newspaper. It may be necessary to correct the techniques of playing golf or tennis. Playing certain musical instruments can strain and so can some crafts: knitting, cutting materials, sewing by hand, or painting pictures. People must always try whenever possible to have the arms supported to avoid static muscle tension.

13. THE SCAPULO-COSTAL AREA

The myofascial pain in the scapulo-costal area and the dorsal column is normally caused by poor posture, tension, and overload of the arms. Osteoarthritis may be present but usually does not cause pain; the pain comes mainly from the soft tissues. You should always make a differential diagnosis and rule out infections, tumours, and inflammatory diseases. A typical diagnosis is scapulo-costal syndrome.

Causes and Mechanisms

Sitting in awkward positions or static jobs may irritate the muscles. It is common to have painful inter-spinous ligaments, with movement restrictions in vertebrae T2 to T8 as increased kyphosis. Driving the car with extended arms causes a static tension that activates trigger points. Another possible cause is holding the phone between the shoulder and the ear. The same tension occurs when you tense your arms while working with the computer mouse or hold newspapers, books or crafts in your arms. In this area, the scapula is kept in place by the muscles. The levator scapulae and rhomboid muscles have to support a lot of stress. These are the muscles that we usually tighten when we get nervous and tense. Beneath the last mentioned muscles, there is still the erector spinae muscle. There are some neurological causes of pain in this area, but they have a different treatment. Heavy rucksacks can cause supra-scapular nerve compression, and cervical radiculitis pain can radiate to the upper part of this area.

Picture:

Usual trigger points in this area:

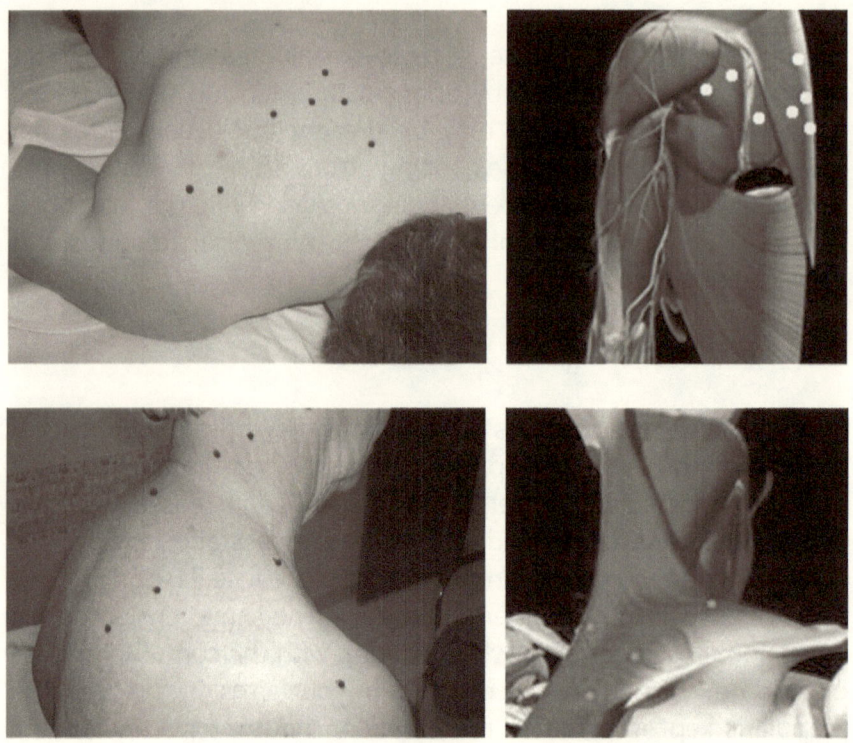

Anatomical images: univadis / 3D Anatomiamalli,
Copyright © Primal Pictures Ltd.

Near the upper medial corner of the scapula, where the levator scapulae muscle is attached, you can sometimes find a heavily scarred, hard, and sore muscle lump because of the great overload this muscle must tolerate. The levator muscle is located under the trapezius muscle, and together they form an inseparable block. The greater rhomboid muscle also has several trigger points. You should also try to palpate the area behind and under the medial scapular border; the serratus anterior muscle is difficult to reach but is sometimes the cause of a very deep pain underneath the shoulder blade. It is best to access this muscle by having the patient face down and bend his arm behind his back. The edge of the scapula is then lifted a little in this position, and the therapist can reach a bit further. The subscapularis muscle has better access from the axilla. The muscle that covers the costo-vertebral joints is called the erector spinae. Here in the picture, is a patient with multiple points in the area of the erector spinae, and the deep layers of the paravertebral muscles. With his spine deformity, his muscles are constantly overloaded, and the patient needs periodical maintenance treatments because this deformity itself cannot be cured.

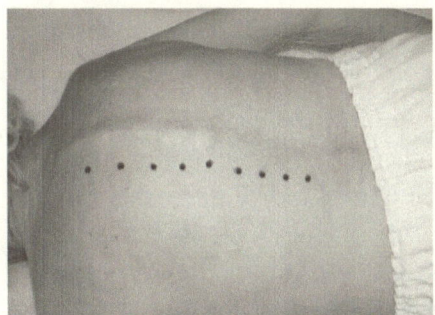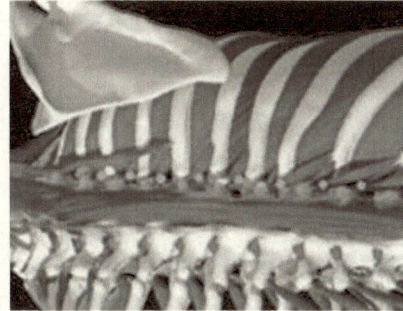

Univadis/3D Anatomiamalli,
Copyright © Primal Pictures Ltd

Finally we have a group of muscles on the scapula, the infraspinatus, and the teres major and teres minor muscles. In these muscles it is very common to find passive and active trigger points. The pain of these muscles often radiate down the arm, and trigger point pain can be confused with a radicular pain.

The Clinical Examination

Begin with the inspection to see if there is asymmetry, muscular atrophy, or misalignment of the spine. The patient can indicate the areas where it hurts, as well as painful movements or positions. Then proceed to palpate and look for contractures and sore spots. If breathing deeply hurts, you have to consider possible pulmonary causes.

You examine whether there is increased sensitivity in the vertebrae by percussion and the springing test, which finds sensitivities in the vertebrae and also examines their mobility. To find radicular nerve pain, it is necessary to examine the cervical spine and muscle function and see if there is any weakness or alterations in the sensitivity. The weakness in arm abduction or external rotation of the Humerus indicates problems with the supra-scapular nerve. The test in which the patient pushes the wall in front with their hands is to see the strength of the rhomboids and the state of the dorsal scapular nerve.

The Treatment

Treatment of trigger points with infiltration of normally 0.2 per cent lidocaine, with 1-2 ml at each point. If you cannot infiltrate, it is good to use the dry needling method. Before the manual treatment, in order to increase the efficiency, it is advisable to use some apparatus that helps the relaxation, decreases pain, and increases the circulation; then proceed to the deep massage of the trigger points and the contracted muscle by gradually increasing the pressure, depending on the tolerance of the patient. Depending on the size of the surface to be treated, the duration of the manual treatment can vary between fifteen and thirty minutes. As always, you have to space out the sessions so that the tissues have recovered from the previous treatment. Soreness can last between one and three days; if it lasts longer, the treatment was too heavy. When the points are very inflamed and there is continuous ache, it is beneficial to use corticosteroid infiltration, and to avoid massage in the first session.

The principle of resting the painful muscles and other tissues is always applied. The overstrained muscles need rest and no exercise. During the treatment sessions, the patient is instructed to perform stretching exercises that help to relax the muscles and their maintenance.

If the spinal column is very rigid, it is convenient to manipulate the vertebras and liberate their movement. For maintenance, there exists auto-manipulation techniques. The patient can press his back against a tennis ball. Stretching the back and hanging on the arms is also good for the back and posture.

Ergonomics and Posture

Analyse the postures of the patient and the possible causes of the painful condition in order to prevent relapses. The patient should be instructed on ergonomics and good posture with the shoulders and arms relaxed, especially in sedentary jobs such as computers or driving a car. It is important to avoid static and tense muscle work. It's good to have breaks in the work and to do some exercises during the breaks. It is often easy to fall into old habits and forget about good posture and relaxing. We can again use simple biofeedback methods to make the patient more conscious and to help him in the correction. Against the tension of the shoulders, you can use an adhesive tape glued to the skin, as mentioned in chapter 11. Against the sinking of the spine, called kyphosing, you can use the clavicular support that stretches the shoulders back and maintains good posture until it becomes automatic.

14. LOW BACK PAIN AND SCIATICA

Lumbalgia is the medical name for lower back pain; sciatica simply means a pain that radiates down the leg. The first thing we distinguish is to see whether the pain is caused by compression of the sciatic nerves, or whether there are other causes. The nerve compression by a prolapsed disc or slipped vertebrae, or by spinal canal stenosis, has a different treatment from myofascial pain.

Doctors and specialists rely too much on modern imaging equipment—they have almost completely forgotten the art of palpation and the different tests for mobility and muscle strength, which are the only way of discovering ill muscles and tendons. Painful contractures and trigger points do not show on an MRI or other scanners

There are too many errors in the diagnosis of the back. It is sadly typical that in many cases, the doctor has not even touched the patient; he is content with images and prescribes medicines or surgery as the only treatment. One sad example is the patient who had six operations on her back, which resulted in equal or worse pain than before the surgery. This lasted more than twenty years after her first operation! The cause of the pain was muscular and easy treatable with the methods that I describe in this book. Have surgeons forgotten about the existence of the muscles? There is a black hole in our preparation at the universities where medicine is taught.

Furthermore, it is forgotten that in perfectly healthy people, there are often changes in the spine due to different degrees of osteoarthritis or herniated discs, which are completely asymptomatic. A herniated disc or arthrosis does not mean that the patient must have pain, just as the patient can often have a lot of pain without any visible pathology in the images. Myofascial pain is far more common than other diseases, and luckily there are these lesser known but effective treatments.

The Causes and Mechanisms

The causes of back pain with and without radiation to the lower extremities are varied. The back has to support a lot, such as overloads and especially the sedentary lifestyle of our times, as well as also many incorrect postures. A healthy spine relies heavily on the movements of the body. The motion pumps the fluids around in the muscles and tissues, which brings nourishment and removes metabolites. Incorrect posture loads the tissues in a non-physiological manner. Unfortunately, we learn poor posture and bad habits in our childhood. Physical education in schools should pay more attention to posture and ergonomics, and how to use the body correctly.

The back can also suffer accidental injuries. Minor injuries normally cause damage to the soft tissue, but severe accidents can cause fractures as well. An MRI scan can detect lesions of the soft structures, especially in the acute phase when the tissues are inflamed.

Stress can also increase muscle tension in any area of the back. As we know, the tension and the static muscle work is gradually activating trigger points and causing damage to the intervertebral discs, with the increased pressure from tight muscles.

Classic causes of back pain are lifting heavy loads with poor technique, and overload in general. For example, moving furniture or carrying heavy bags on a trip, when your normal work is in an office, is an example of the atrocities people do. One must be prepared if doing heavy work such as construction. I sometimes see a patient with a weak body constitution doing a job that requires a body of a weightlifter, and I have to tell them to change jobs. Tension while driving a car is another asymmetric and static overload, as is dragging a golf bag always with the same arm.

Our poor university education, especially related to the spine, results in diagnoses that can almost be anything and have nothing to do with the real causes of pain. Unfortunately, there is a lot of confusion between an authentic sciatica caused by a pinched nerve from a prolapsed disc and with the so-called pseudo sciatica, caused by myofascial trigger points that have often been formed in all the muscles along the pain path (buttock, thigh, calf).

Back pain is a serious concern to the patient. Anxiety causes tension, which then aggravates the situation. The patient begins to be overly careful and avoids pain by tensing the muscles, and this causes a vicious circle. About 80-90 per cent of prolapsed discs heal on their own; the time for healing is usually three to four months, and after this time the prolapse is usually no longer the cause of pain.

The Examination

The examination must be thorough. Start with an examination where the patient is standing up, and notice the deviations from a correct posture. The patient then shows the painful movements. The important thing is to distinguish the pain of myofascial origin from other diseases. It is important to examine the circulation of the legs. The neurological examination is very important: the Laseque test, the deep reflexes, and the skin sensitivity of the different sciatic nerves with the muscle strength are the keys to the distinction between neuropathic and other pain. In most cases the prolapsed intervertebral disc with compression of a nerve is easily diagnosed with these clinical tests, without any imaging studies.

There are other possible causes for nerve entrapment that are less common, such as when the piriformis muscle compresses the sciatic nerve. The femoral cutaneous branches can become trapped in the inguinal canal. The diagnosis of the latter condition is called meralgia paresthetica and is usually solved with a few infiltrations. Interestingly, the sciatica type pain caused by trigger points can mimic the nerve compression pain and gives frequent misdiagnosis. The compressed nerve pains have a completely different treatment than myofascial pain!

The entire course of sciatic pain can be plagued with active myofascial points, and you have to palpate all the muscles of the legs (see last photo). The hip muscles are often the cause of sciatica. In the gluteal area, a few painful points are usually five to nine centimetres deep at the bottom of the muscle layer. Pain of the muscles of the glutei and the sacroiliac area can radiate in a way that the patient thinks is a lower back problem. You can have radiation towards the centre (lower back), or radiation towards the leg as sciatica.

The diagnostic local anaesthesia is very helpful when we are examining the tissues which are causing the pain. Point by point is anesthetized, and you notice the effect on the pain. When the right tissue is anesthetized, the pain disappears or at least diminishes. The Springing test helps to find pain from the deep structures such as the intervertebral discs, and it also evaluates the mobility of each segment. This test should be performed before and after anesthetizing the sore spots.

The lower back has many muscles and ligaments: The inter-spinous ligament is often inflamed—do not forget to palpate these ligaments! The inter-spinous ligament is sometimes the only cause of acute low back pain, and it almost miraculously heals with a small infiltration.

There are several layers of back muscles. The larger or more superficial muscles are the longissimus dorsi, the sacrospinalis, the latissimus dorsi, and the iliocostalis lumborum muscles. Underneath are the multifidus, the semispinalis, the costal levators, the long and short rotators, and even the small inter-spinal muscles. The back has fairly complicated anatomy. The trigger points can be found in any of these structures, and when we palpate, we always try to estimate the depth of the painful tissue. In the photos I've marked some of the most typical points. The location varies somewhat from one patient to another.

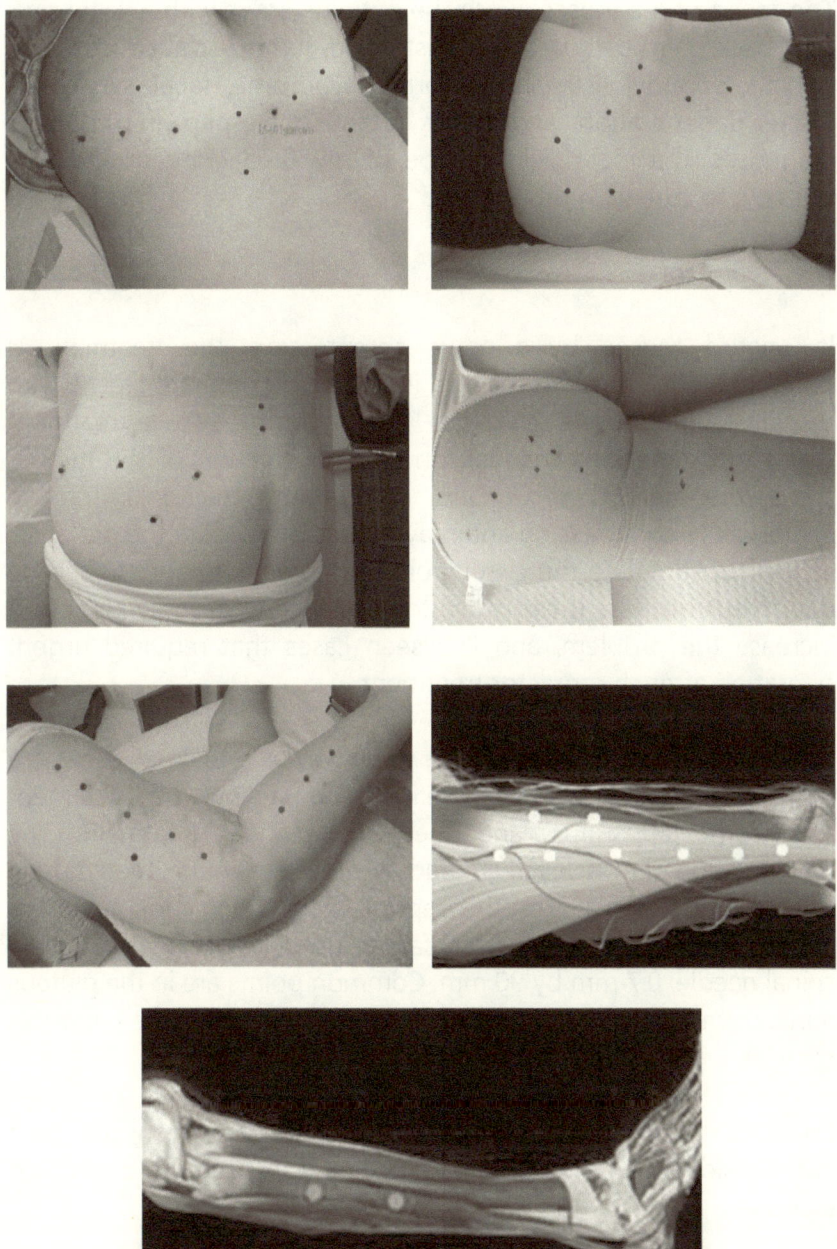

Images anatomical univadis / 3D Anatomiamalli,
Copyright © Primal Pictures Ltd.

The range of diagnoses which the patients arrive with is extensive: Low back pain, osteoarthritis, distortion, lumbo-sciatica, coxalgia, bursitis, spondylolisthesis, piriformis syndrome, facet syndrome, discus degeneration, and discus prolapse. Despite any of these diagnoses, the main pain can be of myofascial origin, and it is possible to cure with this method.

The Treatment

In sciatica caused by a nerve compression, the treatment is different. The most effective is usually complete rest, with painkillers and muscle relaxants. The only form of active treatment that I recommend is manual longitudinal traction of the lumbar spine (the method of Dr Lind, called "auto traction"). Traction opposes the compression and may reduce or relocate the prolapse, as well as stimulate the circulation. Chiropractic treatment can be dangerous because it can move the prolapse to a worse place and increase the problem, and I've seen cases that required urgent operation after chiropractor treatment.

The myofascial pain is treated the same way as explained elsewhere in this book. First you should use infiltration, followed by treatment with some apparatus, and then the manual treatment. The manipulation of muscles must gradually reach even the deep muscle layers—in the gluteal area, the depth is eight to ten centimetre! For infiltration in this area, it is necessary to use a longer needle. I use a spinal needle, 0.7 mm by 90 mm. Common points are in the gluteus minimus muscle, the area of the gemelli, the obturator, the piriformis muscles, and the sacro-tuberous ligament.

Exercises to strengthen the muscles can start when the pain has subsided, but not before. The first exercises are stretching exercises.

Ergonomics and the Posture

The correct use of the back, the working postures, and the correct lifting technique are very important. The pressure to the intervertebral discs is much bigger in an incorrect lift, and turns with a heavy load are dangerous.

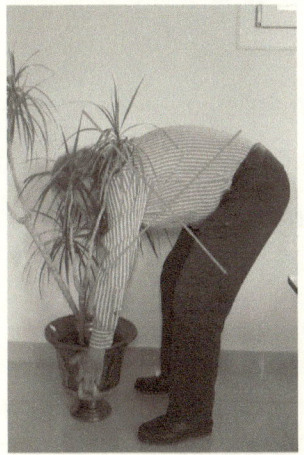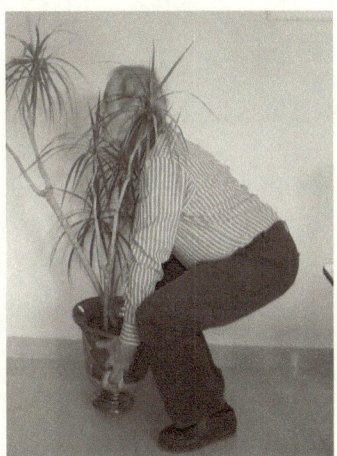

The correct postures of sitting, standing, and walking are as important as the pain treatment itself.

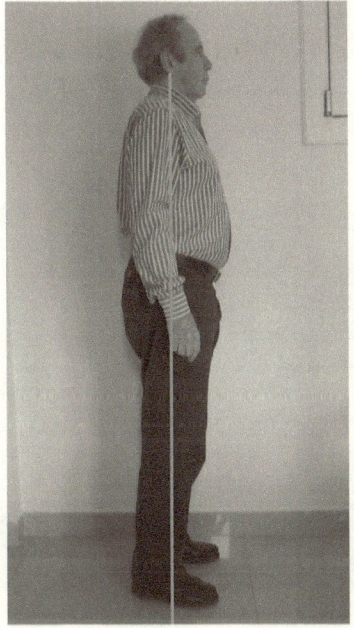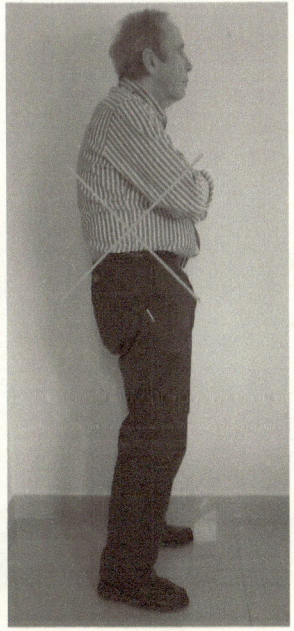

The correction of the posture of the back starts from the knees and then the antero-posterior pelvic tilt. You must also note whether the legs differ in length, which causes a scoliosis that must be corrected.

A common cause, especially in women, is poor work ergonomics in the kitchen. If the work surface is too low, it forces to a bad forward bent position with static tension of the muscles. This can be helped by a small pair of steps that removes a part of the load. Driving a car with a seat that is not suited for the driver causes static tensions, especially in the accelerator leg.

The sitting posture is very important. You have to sit on the ischial tuberosity. If you are half lying on a sofa without support to the lower back, it causes a prolonged stretch to the interspinous ligaments and irritates them. (See the picture below and chapter 8.)

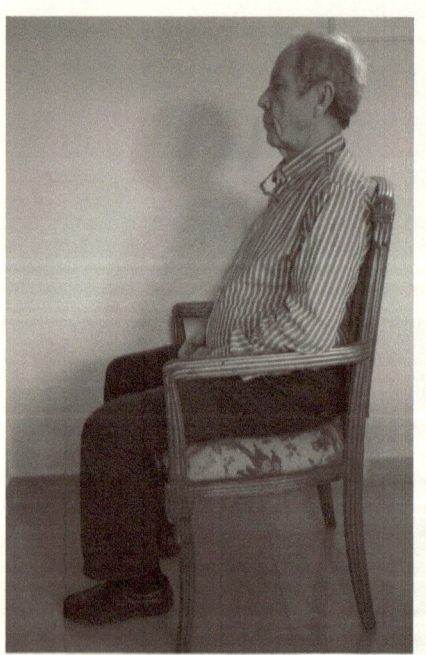
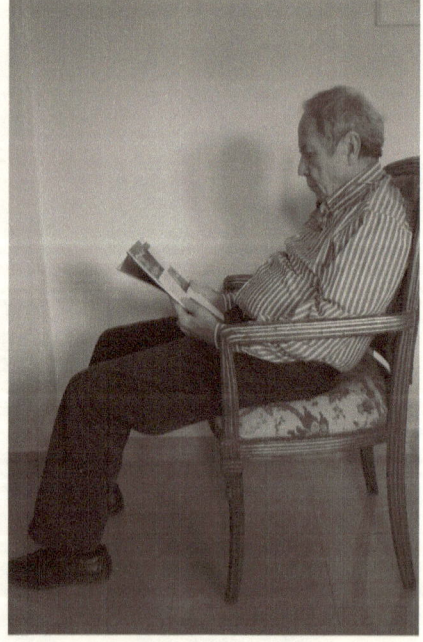

It is very important to have a decent bed to maintain a healthy back. Recent scientific studies have concluded that the most suitable bed is firm and medium soft.

The correct techniques in the gym and different sports are equally important. It is important to ask a trained instructor for the correct performance of all exercise.

15. THE GROIN

Part of the pain of the hip may be at the front in the groin area. The pain is felt especially when you get up from a low chair or try to get out of a car. These pains are often mistaken as the osteoarthritic pain of the hip.

The trigger points may be in the iliopsoas muscle, which flexes the hip and helps in maintaining the erect posture, and also in the pectineus, adductor longus, and gracilis muscles. Much of the iliopsoas is on the inside of the pelvic bone, which is difficult to reach. One can massage only the iliac part; the psoas can be treated with injections in special pain units.

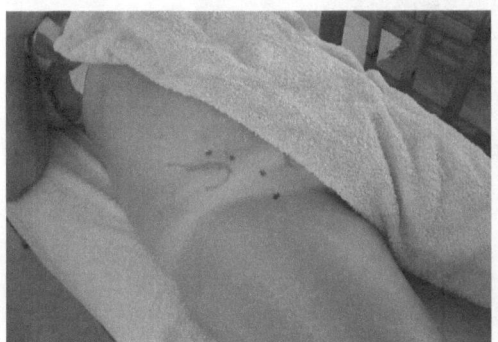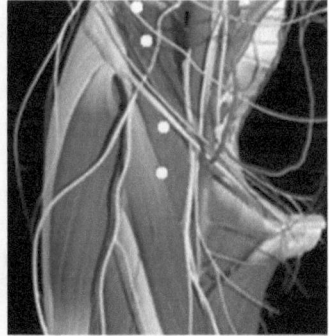

Image Anatomical univadis / 3D Anatomiamalli,
Copyright © Primal Pictures Ltd.

The Causes

One of the most common causes for the iliopsoas muscle is poor posture: when you stand and let the pelvis move forward, or have your arms crossed in front of the chest.

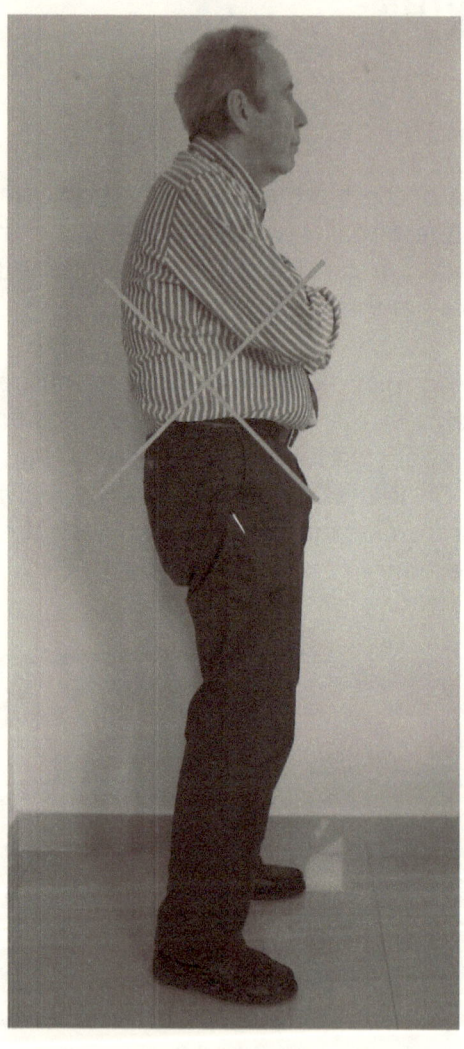

In this position, the iliopsoas muscle is tense. Sitting too long (driving a car) with the hip bent at a sharp angle causes a shortening of the muscle and can also activate trigger points. The tensing of the leg while driving can be another activator, as well as practising sports and other similar situations where you might overstrain these muscles. Sprains of the muscles in a sudden stretch or walking tensely because of some foot pain can trigger on pain in this region.

Pectineus and adductor muscles are overloaded when you sit and press the knees together. Horseback riding is one example. The meralgia paresthetica can cause confusion. It is an entrapment of the lateral femoral cutaneous nerve, and you have to look for hypo—or hyperesthesia in the area of the thigh in order to diagnose this condition

The Treatment

The treatment is done in supine position. The adductor muscles are then more relaxed for treatment, lying on the same side with the other hip flexed and the thigh supported on a firm pillow. The points are then infiltrated and the muscles massaged. The patient is taught stretching exercises for these muscles and should practice them at home daily. As always, try to discover the causes and correct them when possible.

16. THE HIP

The hip is a frequent area of pain. The existing signs of arthritis are often blamed for the pain, and the soft tissues, which are much more likely to be the cause, are forgotten. I repeat here that osteoarthritis causes pain only when it is quite severe. Upon treating the soft tissues, the pain usually is cured. (The osteoarthritis is not altered.)

Other diagnoses that are commonly used in this area include hip bursitis, sciatica, piriformis syndrome, and arthritis of the sacro-iliac joint.

The Causes

The causes are similar to sciatica. Postures that cause prolonged tension in muscles and tendons, or overstraining with heavy loads. Some examples include hanging on the hip while standing, tensing when driving the car, crossing your legs when sitting, and pulling a golf bag always on the same side. The prolonged tension is more harmful than a momentary overload. Often there is a limitation of movements, especially in the rotation, because the muscles are contracted. They have never been stretched to maintain the flexibility or the range of mobility.

The Examination

It is important to test the mobility and notice which movements are causing pain. Ask the patient where he exactly feels the pain. The most common sites of pain in this area are the medial area, near the attachment points of the adductor longus, and the pectineus muscles. At the front side, it can include the points of the groin (see chapter 15). In the lateral area, usually it's the points over the greater trochanter and the gluteus medius muscle. You can also find painful contractures in all the other gluteal muscles.

The sacro-tuberous ligament, the piriformis, and the geminis muscles can have trigger points.

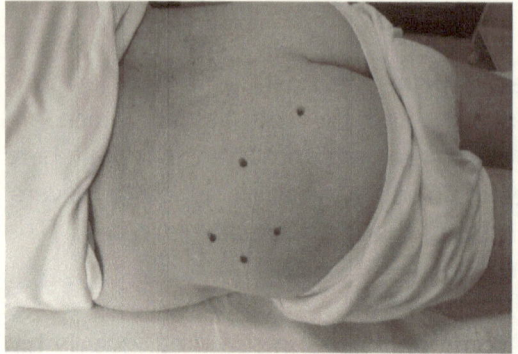
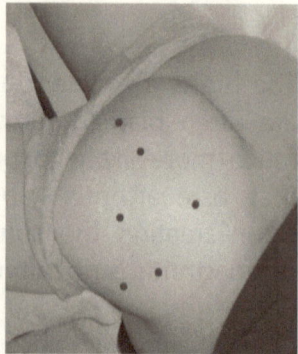

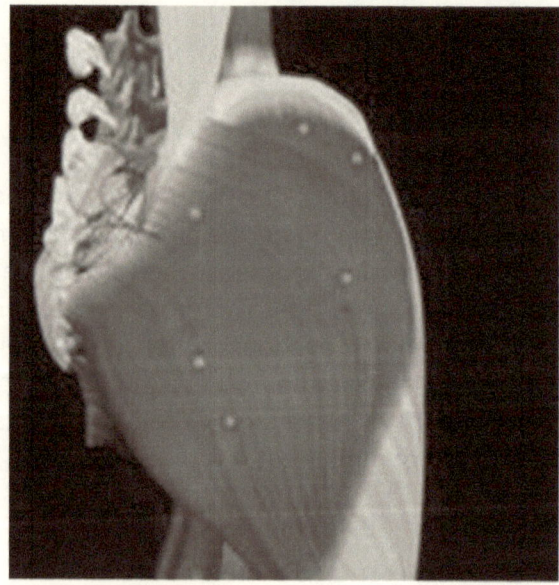

Image Anatomical univadis / 3D Anatomiamalli,
Copyright © Primal Pictures Ltd.

We must realize that this area is very deep and that the points can be found at a depth of eight to ten centimetres. To inject, I use a spinal needle of 0.6 mm by 90 mm. For the massage, it may be necessary to use the elbow in order to get enough strength; the strength must be increased gradually as tolerated by the patient.

The Treatment

The treatment includes infiltrations, the apparatus mentioned before, massage, and stretching. There should also be daily stretching at home, and finally correction of the posture and the ergonomics.

17. THE THIGH

Pains of the upper thigh may be caused by local trigger points or by referred pain. Referred pain usually comes from structures which are close to the thigh, such as the iliac and psoas muscles, very often the buttocks, and sometimes even the lower back. The search for trigger points must be extended to include these areas.

The Causes and Mechanisms

The causes of the activation of trigger points in this area might be the result of a traumatic strain with a fall or overstrain. Overstrain is often chronic and may be from training too hard, wrong postures that cause prolonged tension and reduce the circulation within the muscles, and the habit of usually supporting our body on the same leg whilst standing. Driving a car can create some tension, especially in the accelerator leg. The habit of crossing your legs while sitting also creates tension in the lateral part of the thigh. It is very common to find painful points in the middle and close to the knee; in these cases the patient usually complains of pain in the knee.

In the thigh area, we can sometimes also find neuralgic pain, such as from the sciatic nerve impingement by a discus prolapse. Another area, although rare, is the compression of the lateral cutaneous nerves, passing through the groin ligament—the so-called meralgia paresthetica.

The Examination

As always, carry out a general thorough medical examination to exclude other type of diseases. In this area, it is important to do a neurologic exam in order to distinguish the authentic sciatica caused by a discus prolapse from the pain of myofascial origin, and also meralgia paresthetica. You test for painful and restricted movements and then examine the muscular strength and possible atrophies. Proceed to carry out palpation of the various muscles. The painful points can be located in any of the muscles. Very frequent are the points in the sideline, the vastus lateralis of the rectus femoris muscle (see image).

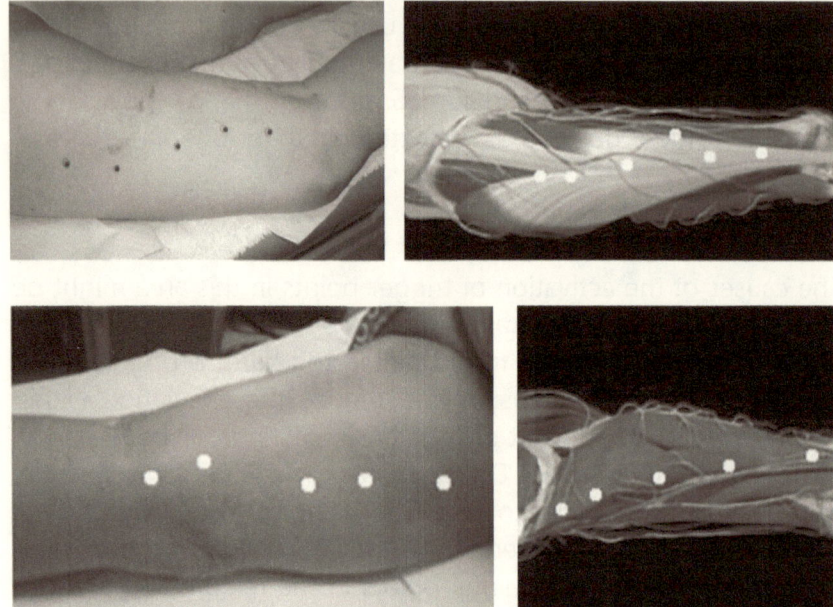

Image Anatomical univadis / 3D Anatomiamalli,
Copyright © Primal Pictures Ltd.

On the medial side, the points often follow the sartorius and adductor muscles from the knee to the hamstring condyle (bottom image). Remember that a part of the medial and lateral muscles are fixed distally below the knee joint, and you have to treat the whole functional unit. On the lateral side, there are often points close to the tendon (and bursa) over the greater trochanter, and even higher up in the lateral gluteus muscles.

In the proximal part of the adductors, there are points very close to the hamstring condyle. At the front side of the thigh, the pain may be a radiation from the ileopsoas trigger points, and the points that lie on the abdominal side of the iliac spine and in the pelvic cavity. The deep psoas muscle, which is located at the sides of the lumbar vertebrae in the abdominal cavity, cannot be reached through massage. The pain at the backside may come from the sciatic nerve or from trigger points in the hamstring muscles.

Even if sciatica is caused by intervertebral discus prolapse, it is important to remember that it often coexists with myofascial trigger points, and treating the muscle pains often alleviates a part of or all of the pain.

The Treatment

To treat the muscles, they have to be totally relaxed. It is better to treat each side at a time, rotating the body and holding the leg, as seen in the companion videos. The treatment postures for the different areas are also important for accessibility to points deep in the groin, or the points of the iliopsoas muscle.

Infiltrate the sore points and then apply the adjuvant treatment with an apparatus; then carry out the deep massage techniques to relax the muscles and to inactivate the existing trigger points. Afterwards, teach the patient the stretching exercises for the tight, contracted muscles, which he must also do at home. The most commonly shortened muscles are the adductor and knee flexor muscles, as well as the hamstrings and the iliopsoas.

The Ergonomics

Give instructions for better posture and the proper ergonomics to prevent relapse.

18. THE KNEE

Knee pain is very common. A common mistake is to blame existing osteoarthritis for the pain.; Almost everyone after a certain age has some osteoarthrosis. This belief is totally wrong! It is sad that so many people suffer needlessly from chronic pain and have to burden their body with different drugs. Everyone who has pain in the knee should be examined (and treated) for the trigger points. My treatment can alleviate (and sometimes remove) the pain and inflammation, restoring the function in spite of the existing osteoarthritis (when there is still some cartilage left at the joint surface). Treatment often even alleviates the pain of rheumatoid arthritis. In the extremely advanced arthrosis, when there is no cartilage left, surgical replacement of the joint is the only solution.

Many sports can easily cause more or less serious lesions in the structures of the knee. With this method, you can accelerate the healing process of trauma. The knee is often exposed to minor trauma and overload, even in people who do not participate in any sports. Excess body weight also puts a strain on the knee.

The joint is solely covered by the medial sartorius muscle; the rest of the covering structures are tendons and the joint capsule. The tendons as well as the muscles develop trigger points, which should be equally treated. It is very common to find painful points in the patellar ligament and the lateral retinaculum, such as in the proximal pole of the patella in the attachment of the rectus femoris muscle. The patient might feel, as a knee pain, even the pain originating from the muscles that are close to the knee.

The Causes

If people start walking much more than usual, it can inflame the knee or worse, if the terrain is mountainous or there are many stairs. Also, prolonged relative overstrain can gradually irritate the tissues (mounting bicycle, tennis, jogging, etc.). Tensions from awkward postures can also activate trigger points. Another common cause is the small sprains that occur many times, even without being conscious of it. A wrong walking habit, rotating the feet outwards, gives small jerks to the inner ligaments. Foot problems like a flat foot, where the foot sinks at the inside and consequently stretches the ligaments at the inside of the knee, can also cause issues. Some traumas, like a fall with a sprain, can leave a chronic pain when the tissue does not heal correctly.

Examination and Diagnosis

The patient's history and descriptions of the exact location of pain and of the painful movements help to find the affected tissues. The examination reveals if there are inflamed tissues or excess of intra-articular fluid. Test skin temperature: an increase is a sign of infection or inflammation, and a decrease might be the sign of a circulatory problem. Stability of the joint must be studied to find ruptured ligaments. Carry out tests to find meniscal injuries, and if necessary, do an MRI scan. Do not forget the use of the diagnostic local anaesthesia in doubtful cases! Analyse the mechanics of walking and possible abnormal forces affecting the knee to try to correct the causes.

To assess the extent and impact of osteoarthritis, a conventional radiography is enough. In a large majority of cases of knee pain, the pain is due to the painful ligaments and their corresponding muscles. Any tendon can be affected, even the coronary ligament, but there are common points. The points can be more accurately located with a round-ended stick (the finger is too thick for some points). The images give examples of possible locations of the tender points.

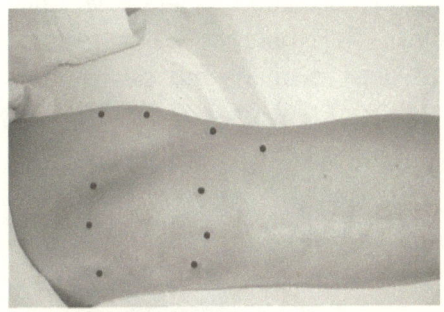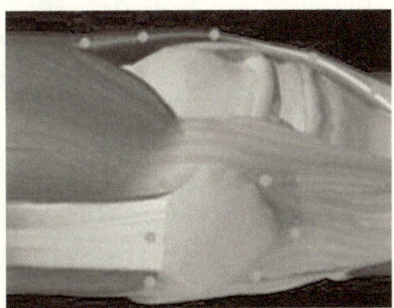

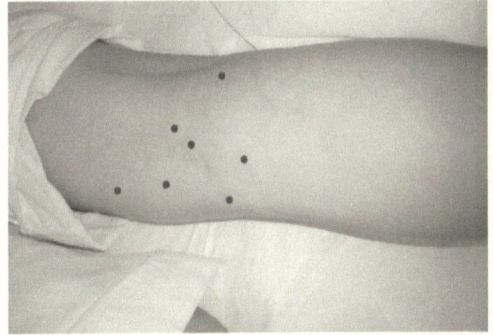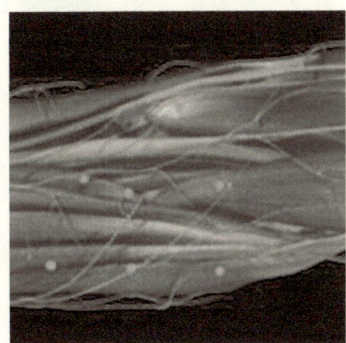

Image Anatomical univadis / 3D Anatomiamalli,
Copyright © Primal Pictures Ltd.

The Treatment

The trigger points of the knee need smaller amounts of liquid (0.5-1.0 cc) to be infiltrated. One ligament can have multiple tender points. A majority of the time it is convenient to use a small amount of cortisone. Massage is also an important part in the treatment of the ligaments (for the massage techniques, view the companion videos.) Resting the knee is an especially important part of the treatment, and the patient should avoid doing things that are painful. Every time the knee hurts, it irritates the affected tissue and prolongs the healing. However, it is often difficult to get the patient to rest sufficiently.

To achieve permanent results, the therapist must try to find out and correct the causes. Care must be taken to correct the possible orthopaedic problems and any gait problems. There exist specialists who do gait analysis and correction. Check that the patient wears appropriate footwear. The therapist must correct all postures that cause prolonged tension of the muscles or the tendons.

19. THE CALF

Calf pains are quite common; they can occur alone or be part of sciatica. The calf is a common place for night cramps, which may be the product of poor metabolism of the muscles in this area. Achilles tendinitis is also an overload of this area, and the entire functional unit should be treated. (Attention: quinolone antibiotics can cause tendinitis and even rupture the Achilles tendon.) Blood circulation problems—arterial, venous, or lymphatic—can also cause pain and discomfort in the calf. More rare is the entrapment of local peripheral nerves. Any tissue with poor circulation and metabolism will, sooner or later, interfere and give symptoms.

The Causes

There are many causes: training too hard, walking (uphill), running, dancing, cycling without proper care of the muscles such as stretching, warming up, and massage. The muscles and tendons can become affected from static tension, standing still for long periods of time, driving long distances in a car, or sitting and leaning your feet solely on the ball of the feet (often a nervous habit).

The Examination

Do a complete medical check-up to rule out diseases that are not myofascial. Use a visual examination: skin colour, swellings, deformities, atrophy, and varicose veins. Touch the skin to feel the temperature, arterial pulses, and type of oedema or chronic cellulitis. Palpate the tissues to find sore and hardened tissue areas. A clinical neurological examination is important to rule out pain of nervous origin. In the picture, I have marked the most common location of painful points.

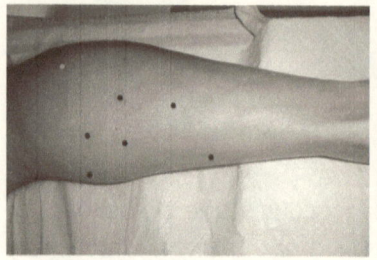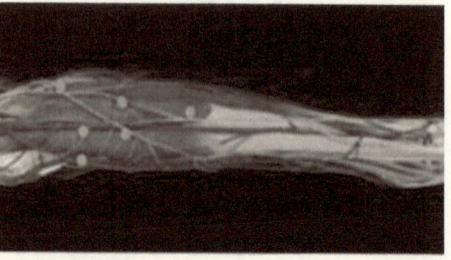

Imagen anatómico: Univadis / 3D Anatomiamalli,
Copyright © Primal Pictures Ltd.

The Treatment

This treatment aims to restore the circulation and the metabolism in the tissues, and it is effective in most cases. Begin with infiltrating the trigger points with local diluted anaesthetic, as usual (video). Massage until you achieve the relaxation of the muscles. The cramps are more frequent when the muscle metabolism is impaired by trigger points, but it may also have other causes, such as lack of magnesium, a lack of fluid (water), and a lack of vitamin B12. The massage must press the muscles against the bone to be effective. The calf muscle tends to slide to either side, and the effectiveness of the massage is lost. (It also happens easily with the biceps muscle of the upper arm, which is rather elusive.) See the video "Treatment of the Achilles Tendon".

Other Pains

The pain when the arterial supply fails is called claudication, and it occurs when the arteries are clogged and calcified and their flow is reduced, causing pain especially when walking. Even in these cases, this treatment can help. Often, besides the poor arterial circulation, there are coexisting muscular spasms and trigger points. Treating the muscular part of the problem can improve the muscular metabolism and perhaps also the general situation; it can maybe even postpone surgery.

The peronei nerve occasionally gets trapped at the head of the fibular bone. The issue can sometimes be solved with an injection of diluted anaesthetic into the nerve channel, achieving more space and liberating the nerve without surgery. This procedure works for many trapped nerves. I also have good results with treating poor venous-lymphatic circulation. In these cases, the cause is a poor return of liquids. A frequent cause is the insufficiency of the varicose veins. This condition is not a contraindication for massage. Another cause could be a scar after a trauma, venous thrombosis, or an infection such as erysipelas, which causes a chronic cellulitis.

In these cases, the tissue feels hard, immobile, and oedematous. You cannot easily distinguish the different tissues by palpating; everything feels like a hard block. The pigmentation may also be increased (because of the poor metabolism), and there might be ulcers of different sizes and depths. The treatment of these cases are complicated and can take time, but it is possible to achieve great improvement. Because of the large sensitivity of the leg in these cases, and because of the hardness of this tissue, the manual treatment must be quite strong. In order to soften the scar tissue, use a more concentrated anaesthetic (0.5-1 per cent) to allow the patient to be more comfortable while you work. Many times the hardness of the tissue is such that it takes a lot of force to infiltrate and press in the liquid. Use a smaller syringe in order to increase the pressure enough, and be sure to infiltrate all the hardened tissue. Then, using manual techniques (connective tissue massage), soften the hardness and improve the impaired circulation.

Lymphatic-circulatory massage is used to propel the fluids. The pinching technique (connective tissue massage) is used to loosen the scar tissue and help the healing.

Never massage infected tissues, or when there is an acute thrombophlebitis! The often present and persistent oedema in these legs is not a good thing. Pressure builds up in the tissues, and the circulation is further worsened. Try to decrease the swelling by other means, such as diuretic medicines or support stockings.

The Anterolateral Part

Anterolateral refers to the following muscles: tibialis anterior, fibularis, and the long toe extensors. The pain is felt on these muscles and sometimes radiates to the dorsum of the foot. In this area, there may also be neuralgic pain, which must be detected because a different treatment is necessary.

There are numerous causes for sore muscles: prolonged tension when driving a car or tightening these muscles when sitting and supporting only the toes on the floor (sometimes a nervous habit).; wearing shoes with high heels or walking or running incorrectly; ankle trauma, which can activate trigger points in these muscles. The treatment consists of infiltration and massage with the correction of possible causes.

20. THE FOOT AND ANKLE

The foot is subjected to great strain caused by the weight of the body; it is also affected by other important factors such as the use of inappropriate footwear. The foot may have problems and pain from poor circulation or neurological problems, such as diabetic neuropathy or a trapped nerve. The feet influence other parts of the body, up to the back. Trigger points located much higher up on the leg and the thigh may also radiate to the foot. Furthermore, look for points outside the area where the pain is concentrated. The foot has many small muscles that can be overstrained. Do not forget the inter-osseous muscles because they are often sore.

Some different diagnoses used by practitioners for foot pain are osteoarthritis, tendinitis of the Achilles tendon, sesamoiditis, Morton's foot, plantar fasciitis, heel spur, and inflammation of ligaments and tendons (trauma or overload). In most of these conditions, activation of trigger points is an important part of the pain—even the pain of rheumatoid arthritis can be alleviated substantially with this treatment.

The Causes

It is easy to twist the foot on a curb or receive a blow or impact when jumping. Especially if one is practicing certain sports, injuries are common, and so is overstrain. Our daily life has become quite sedentary, and then during the holidays we go sightseeing, visit museums, and go on shopping tours. We spend hours walking or standing, and our feet are protesting with pain. The body is not trained for that kind of strain. We also use inappropriate footwear for this type of marathon, which causes even more strain.

Another cause is walking without shoes. If the foot is used to being in a shoe, the strain is much greater than normal. In principle it is healthy for the foot to walk like this, but the transition must be gradual. Too narrow shoes and shoes with high heels are not good for the feet and can cause pain. Walking in the countryside or the mountains requires different shoes than if one is walking or jogging on a hard surface such as asphalt. If the foot already has some structural changes such as flat foot (over pronation), it tolerates less effort.

The Examination

Clinical history is always important. We are looking for the causes of the condition: how did the pain start? Is there a general disease that could explain the symptoms? The examination of the foot begins with an inspection of how the patient stands. Look for deformities like bunions or decreased natural arches (flat foot). Always observe the patient walking with bare feet. The feet are best examined with a special glass bench with a mirror. The trend of internal rotation is best seen when the patient is standing on one foot only, bending the knee. It is also useful to examine the patient's old shoes for signs of wear. For lasting results, it is vital to correct some of these anatomical changes. The foot may need orthotics or shoes with better cushioning and more support, and sometimes even surgical operations (bunions, hammertoes, etc.).

Continue with a systematic review: check the appearance of skin such as redness (gout or infection), wounds, or callosities. Is there oedema, and is it local or more generalized? Then go on to examine the arterial and venous circulation. Check the nervous system for paraesthesia, hyperesthesia, and muscular strength and jerk reflexes. Be sure to look at the mobility and function of joints and painful movements.

When these tasks are complete, palpate to locate the trigger points. Sometimes the therapist's finger is too thick for the smaller trigger points of the foot; in that case, use a tester (a round-ended stick). Trigger points can exist in any of the muscles (short extensors, short flexors, short abductors, inter-osseous muscles, the lumbrical muscles, etc.). In addition to the points in the muscles, there are hurting points in tendons, ligaments, and joint capsules.

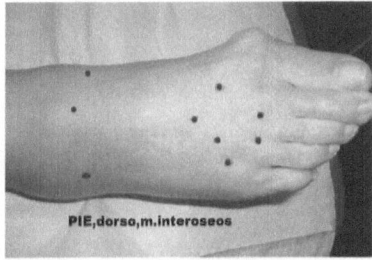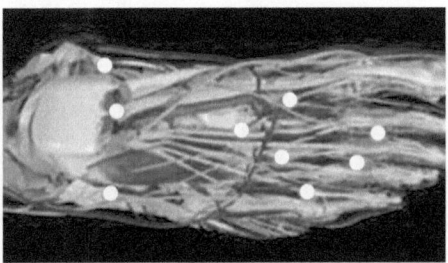

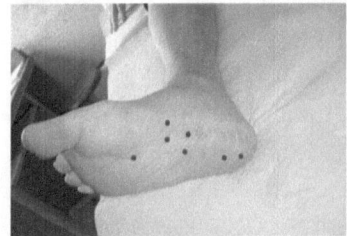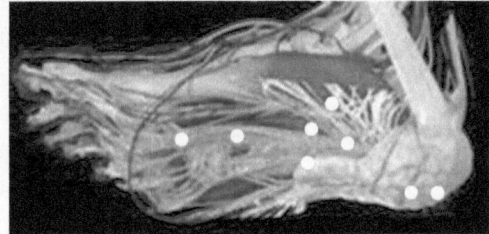

Image Anatomical univadis / 3D Anatomiamalli,
Copyright © Primal Pictures Ltd.

The photo above has the points of a plantar fasciitis and a heel spur; these conditions often coexist.

The Treatment

Deactivation of trigger points: the treatment applies equally to tendon and muscle or joint capsule. The first one infiltrates the painful points. At the foot, the amounts of liquid are much smaller, from 0.1 cc up to 1.0 cc per point. The next step is the adjuvant treatment with some equipments selected by the therapist.

Next, commence the massage, starting with lighter techniques and gradually increasing the pressure for the deeper structures. When there is a lot of inflammation, the massage has to be very light and short in duration; sometimes it is advisable to start the first treatment sessions without massage (only infiltrate, and order rest and possible simultaneous treatment with anti-inflammatory medicines). The Dr Furter technique (video) is helpful. At first, five to ten minutes of massage to a foot may be enough. Manual massage with the fingertips is gentler when there is a lot of pain or inflammation. Treatment of the heal spur also benefits from massage. The massage needs a lot of pressure, so use a stick if necessary. When there is a lot of oedema, use techniques that help the venous and lymphatic circulation and that reduce tissue fluid.

Complete rest or at least relative immobility is necessary to heal irritated and sore tissues. It seems that sometimes the most difficult thing for the patient is to stop walking. Without sufficient rest, one can obstruct any treatment results. It often happens that when the patient gets up in the morning, he feels more pain, which begins to diminish or disappear after walking around a while. When the tissues get warmed up, the patient can continue to walk with less pain. This is misleading—irritated tissues have no chance to heal when they are in use. The use of the foot prolongs the time of healing. Foot orthotics can help the foot, silicone pads can cushion the heel, and there are special shoes like the MBT (Masai Barefoot Technology) shoes that are better at protecting the feet.

To achieve lasting results, it is necessary to correct the possible causes of the problem. The patient should consult a podiatrist to get appropriate shoes with proper orthotic support. Instruct gradual training of the feet, and remove painful corns or warts. In foot trauma, use the necessary support as bandages or even plaster casts. Strapping with inelastic sports tape is a good way to limit unwanted movements during the healing process.

The Ankle

The most frequent problems are sprains of the ankle that are incorrectly cured and Achilles tendinitis. Both are treatable by using the following method. To begin with the ankle, have a thorough medical examination, including possible X-rays, tests of stability and mobility, and examining the circulation and neurological state. The ligaments that are affected more often are the deltoid, the tibionavicular, the talo-fibulare anterius, and the fibulo-calcaneal ligaments.

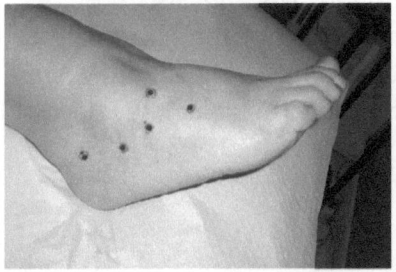 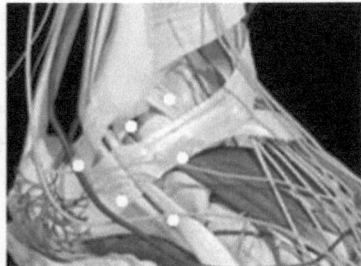

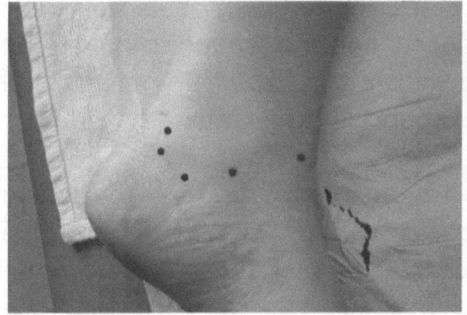 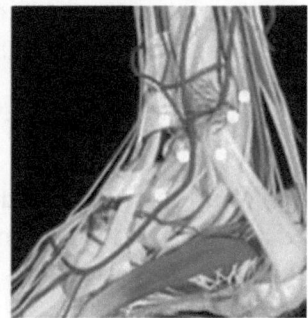

Image Anatomical univadis / 3D Anatomiamalli,
Copyright © Primal Pictures Ltd.

An inflamed tendon or ligament usually has a reaction of swelling around it. (The images of the ankles have almost no visible inflammation left.) The ankle pain points are treated as all other trigger points. The diluted corticosteroid injection is more effective than the anaesthetic alone. The quantities are small, 0.1- 0.5 ml to the individual points.

Also in the ankle, massaging is important because it increases circulation and helps the healing process. The techniques I use are done with my fingers (type Cyriax) or the stick massage (Dr Furter), and I often combine both. It is good to combine lymphatic massage techniques when there is oedema. When the tissue gets warmer with the massage, the pain diminishes, even during the same session.

In a relatively small treatment zone like the ankle, the treatment times are shorter to avoid further irritation. Sessions between five and fifteen minutes are long enough. Healing also requires rest and immobility. Rest is an important part of the treatment. When the inflamed, painful tissues have calmed down, they start to gradually tolerate better use of the foot. The ankle may need some support during healing, to avoid excessive movements.

Achilles Tendinitis

This tendinitis occurs mostly from repeated overloads—for example, in runners. In more chronic cases, the tendon and its surrounding tissues are scarred and hardened, and the tendon is injured more easily. Remember that the overload is in the whole functional unit (all the calf muscles), and it is important to treat the whole unit.

The infiltrations are placed in the hardened tissue at the side and beneath the tendon. In most cases I use a diluted steroid with anaesthetic. Trigger points of the calf muscle itself do not usually require corticosteroids. The massage has to reach the tissues underneath the Achilles tendon and loosen the scarred tissues. To heat up, first I use the Furter technique, and afterwards connective tissue techniques are needed to release the tendon and soften the surrounding tissues. The patient has to do stretching exercises, initially softly, and he also has to have the leg in relative rest.

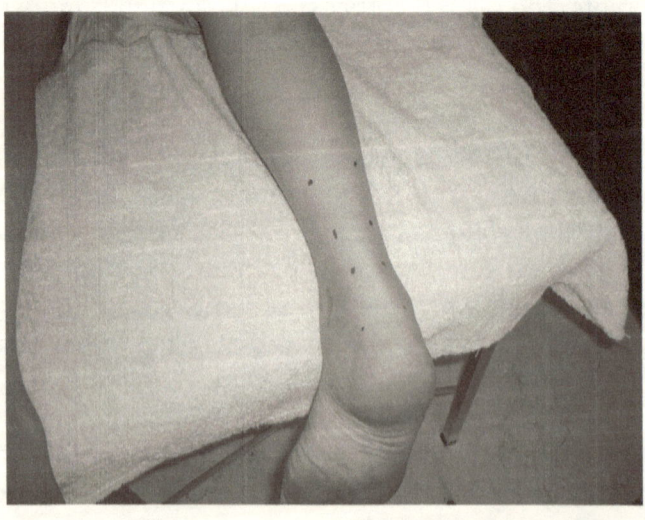

LITERATURE AND SOURCES

G. Ambrose and G. Newbold, *A Handbook of Medical Hypnosis* (London: Baillière Tindall, 1980)

Johannes Asdonk, *Ärtzliche Erfahrung mit der des Krampfaderbeines Lymphdrainage-Massage* (Heidelberg: Karl F. Haug Verlag, 1967)

P.E. Baldry, *Acupuncture Trigger Points and Musculoskeletal Pain.* (UK: Churchill Livingstone, 1989)

J. Bischko, *Einführung in die Akupunktur* (Heidelberg, Haug Verlag, 1970)

Asbjörn Bragstad, *Skuldersmärter og Årsaker til Disse* (Oslo: Informa Geigy, 1977)

Asbjörn Bragstad, *Low Back Pain Syndrome.* (Oslo: Informa geigy, 2/3 1976)

Rene Cailliet, *Low Back Pain (1982), Shoulder pain (1966), Foot and Ankle Pain (1968), Hand Pain and Impairment (1975), Knee Pain and Disability (1973).*(Philadelphia: F.A. Davis Company)

J.H. Cyriax, *Textbook of Orthopaedic Medicine* (Lippincot, Williams & Wilkins, 1969)

Clair Davies,*The Trigger Point Therapy Workbook* (Oakland: New Harbinger Publications, Inc., 2004)

J.P. Dosch, *Lehrbuch der Neuraltherapi nach Hunecke* (Heidelberg, Karl F. Haug Verlag, 1970)

Ejnar Ericsson, *Illustrated Handbook in Local Anaeshesia* (Copenhagen, I.Chr.Sørensen &.CoA/S, 1969)

Olav Evjenth and Jern Hamberg, *Töjning av Muskler II* (Alfta, Alfta Rehab Förlag, 1980)

Hede, Leube,Teirlich, *Grundrisse der Bindegewebsmassage* (Stuttgart, Gustav Fischer Verlag, 1970)

Carl Herman Hjortsjö, *Rörelseapparaten.* (Lund, CWK Gleerups Förlag, 1967)

Freddy M. Kaltenborn, *Manual Mobilization of the Joints: Extremities* (2002) *and Maniual Mobilization of the Joints: The Spine* (Orthopedic Physical Therapy Products, 2012)

Gertrud A.M. Lind, *Auto-Traction Treatment of Low Back Pain and Sciatica* (Linköping, Sturetryckeriet A.B., 1974)

Felix Mann, *Acupuncture (1962)* and *The Meridians of Acupuncture (1964)* and *The Treatment of Disease by Acupuncture(1963)* (London, William Heinemann).

Lyn Marshall, *Yoga* (London, Ward Lock Limited, 1976)

Harris H. McIlwain Harris and Debra Fulghum, *The Fibromyalgia Handbook* (Henry Holt and Company, LLC, 1996)

H.J. Montag and P.D. Asmussen, *Functional Bandaging of the Limbs* (Hamburg, BDF Medical Programm Bibliothek, 1983)

Alf L. Nachemson, *Low Back Pain Etiology and Treatment,*(Journal of Clinical Medicine, Jan. 1971) and *Towards a Better Understanding of Low-Back Pain* (Journal of Rheumatology and Rehabilitation, 1975/14)

Walter Alexander Naddel, *The Slipped Disc and the Aching Back of Man* (Glasgow, J.R. Reid Printers Ltd., 1985)

Lars Peterson and Per Renström, *Sports Injuries Their Prevention and Treatment.* (Mosby, 1986)

Pekka Pöntinen, *Low Level Laser Therapy as a Medical Treatment Modality*.(Tampere, Art Urpo Ltd., 1992)

A.Rodríguez and L.Fernandez and F. Navarro and A.Herrera, *Basis of Medical-Surgical-Musculoskeletal Diseases* (Laboratorios Menarini, 1999)

C. Claus Schnorrenberger, *Das Neue Chen-chiu Heilprinzip* (Freiburg, Aurum Verlag, 1975)

Henrik Seyfarth, *Treatment of Torticollis*,(Acta Neurolgica Scandinavica 1963/39) "Lidocain injktionen in Myos".

Bernie Siegel, *Love, Medicine and Miracles* (William Morrow Paperbacks 1998)

David G.Simons and Janet G. Travell, *Myofascial Pain and Dysfunction* (Lippincott Williams & Wilkins, 1998)

O. Carl Simonton, *Getting Well Again* (Bantam 1992)

Devin Starlanyl, *Fibromyalgia and Chronic Myofascial Pain* (Oakland, New Harbinger Publications Inc., 2001)

Alan Stoddard, *Manual of Osteopathic Practice* (1969) and, *Manual of Osteopathic Treatment* (1959) (London, Hutchinsons Medical Publications)

Sven A. Sölveborn, *The Book About Stretching* (Japan Pubns, 1985)

S. Yesudian and E. Haigh, *Sport + Yoga* (Drei Eichen Verlag 2001)

Steven D.Waldman, *Atlas of Uncommon Pain Syndromes* (Elsevier Science, 2004)

Wu Wei-Ping, *Chinese Acupuncture* (GB, Health Science Press, 1973)

DVD CONTENT

-Introduction 4:57

-Infiltration of a Calf 1:37

-The Achilles Tendon Treatment 2:15

-The Ankle, Lateral 0:49

-The Ankle, Medial 1:22

-The Anterior Tibial Group 1:48

-The Armpit 0:55

-The Biceps 0:50

-The Calcaneus 0:45

-The Calf 1:11

-The Finger Joint 1:13

-The Foot, Dorsal 1:22

-The Foot, Plantar 1.03

-The golfers Elbow 0:52

-The Hip Region 1:10

-The Iliopsoas 0:53

-The Knee, Anterior 1:26

-The Knee, Medial 1:04

-The Knee, Posterior 0:57

-The Lumbar-Gluteal Zone 2:37

-The Neck, Dorsal 0:58

-The Shoulder and Upper Back 1:44

-The Shoulder, Front 1:12

-The Shoulders 1:26

-The Side of the Neck 1:40

-TheTemporo-Mandibular and Scalenus Zone 1:19

-The Tennis Elbow 1:29

-The Thigh, Front 1:14

-The Thigh, Medial 1:24

-The Thigh, Posterior 1:11

-The Forearm 1:11

-The Thumb, Abductors 1:21

-The Treatment of Myofascial Sciatica 1:33

-The Treatment Posture for Sciatica 0:15

-The Underarm

You can download the videos from my website: www.penttiraaste.com